# Secrets of Na~~~~~
# (SONW®)

## Activate the Extraordinary
## Healing Capabilities of Your Body

Irmansyah Effendi, M.Sc.

SECRETS OF NATURAL WALKING®
Activate the Extraordinary Healing Capabilities of Your Body

Copyright ©2018 Irmansyah Effendi, M.Sc.

The information in this book is not to replace physical, medical, or emotional treatments based on physicians' advice. The author provides information based on feedback from various instructors, testimonials from a large number of workshop participants, and his own personal experience and observation. Should readers choose to use the information in this book for themselves, which is their constitutional rights, the author and the publisher assume no responsibility for their actions.

Publisher
Natural Way of Living
P.O. Box 1470
Joondalup DC, WA 6919
Australia
www.naturalwayofliving.com

ISBN: 978-0-9945524-1-9

This book is for general informational purposes only. The material presented is not intended to be a substitute for professional medical advice, diagnosis, or treatment, and does not constitute medical advice. Please consult your physician for personalized medical advice. Always seek the advice of a physician or other qualified healthcare provider with any questions regarding a medical condition. Never disregard or delay seeking professional medical advice or treatment because of something you have read in this book.

It is recommended that you consult your physician prior to starting any new exercise program. Before practicing the skills described in this book, be sure that your environment is suitable for such activity, and do not take risks beyond your level of experience, aptitude, training, and comfort level. The use of any information provided in this book is solely at your own risk, and you are taking full responsibility for your actions and safety.

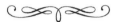

*May we become more grateful to the Creator for our physical body and all other beautiful Gifts of Love from the Creator.*

# Table of Contents

**Preface**

**CHAPTER 1: BENEFITS OF WALKING PROPERLY**  01
The benefits of walking properly explained  02
How can walking give such abundant benefits?  03
For all ages  04
Some experiences after walking properly  05

**CHAPTER 2: THE HUMAN BODY IS A GIFT
OF LOVE FROM OUR CREATOR**  27
The extraordinary repair, growth and natural
healing capabilities  30
Everything functions properly when not disturbed  34
Wounded skin  35
Broken bones  35

**CHAPTER 3: UNDERSTANDING WALKING IS
AKIN TO UNDERSTANDING NUTRITION**  39
Guidelines for a balanced diet (food pyramid)  39
The elements within each step  49

**CHAPTER 4: RELATIONSHIP BETWEEN THE
WAY WE WALK AND OUR HEALTH**  53
Posture, spine and health  53
Research by Dr. Roger Sperry  54

Research by Dr. Henry Winsor                                  55
All systems within the human body are interconnected          64


**CHAPTER 5: COMMON MISTAKES IN WALKING       65**
Even the way we move our legs matters                         65
Finding your ideal distances                                  67
Instructions to evaluate your right foot                      70
Guidelines to evaluate the left leg                           80


**CHAPTER 6: MISTAKES CAUSED BY**
**OTHER FACTORS                                            91**
Footwear                                                     91
Other factors                                               95


**CHAPTER 7: SECRETS OF NATURAL**
**WALKING® (SONW)                                          97**


**CHAPTER 8: BASIC UNDERSTANDING OF**
**SECRETS OF NATURAL WALKING®             101**
Causes of mistakes                                          101
Walking naturally                                           102


**CHAPTER 9: WALKING METHOD IMPROVEMENT**
**AND THE STAGES OF CHANGES TO THE BODY    111**
Changing the way you walk is not difficult                  111
Stages of changes to the body                              113


**CHAPTER 10: BASIC UNDERSTANDING OF**
**NATURAL WALKING                                        119**
Distance between left foot and right foot                   120
Distance between the front foot and the back foot           121
How to place the sole of the foot on the ground            121
Walking has to be straight                                 123

The whole body directed straight forward      123

**CHAPTER 11: 6 BASIC KEYS OF SECRETS OF NATURAL WALKING® (SONW)**      **125**

**CHAPTER 12: KEY 1: SWINGING THE LEG**      **129**
Instructions      129
Explanation      129
Body weight      130

**CHAPTER 13: KEY 2: PUMPING THE PAD OF THE FOOT**      **139**
Instructions      139
Explanation      140
Body weight      141

**CHAPTER 14: KEY 3: GLIDING THE BODY WHILE ROLLING THE BACK FOOT**      **149**
Instructions      149
Explanation      150
Body Weight      150

**CHAPTER 15: KEY 4: LETTING ALL ADJUSTMENTS HAPPEN**      **155**
Instructions      156
Explanation      156
Body weight      157

**CHAPTER 16: KEY 5: LETTING GO THE BODY WEIGHT INTO THE EARTH**      **161**
Instructions      161
Explanation      161
Body weight      162

**CHAPTER 17: KEY 6: THE NEXT STEP**     **165**
Instructions     165
Explanation     165
Body weight     166

**CHAPTER 18: IMPORTANT MATTERS RELATED
TO SECRETS OF NATURAL WALKING® (SONW)**     **169**
Changes require time     169
People who find it challenging to practice SONW     169
People who require a walking stick or other walking
aids to assist in walking     170
Soreness vs. pain and cleansing in SONW     171
Seriously vs. carefully     172
Older people in practicing SONW     172
SONW is nothing special     173
Expression of gratitude to our Creator     173
Taking care of our body as best as possible     174

**CHAPTER 19: NATURAL WALKING IN DAILY LIFE**   **177**
How do we run?     179
How do we walk uphill and downhill on uneven
and steep surfaces?     179
Climbing up the stairs properly     180
Climbing down the stairs properly     181
How do we walk backwards?     182

**CHAPTER 20: DISCOVERY OF SONW**     **183**
Background     183
Formulation     185
Formal workshops     186
The development of SONW     187

**CHAPTER 21: TESTIMONIALS**            **191**

**CHAPTER 22: ADDITIONAL INFORMATION**     **219**

SONW centers            219

Classes at SONW centers            220

Works cited            225

Favourite SONW instructors            226

SONW instructors' contact info            260

Irmansyah Effendi M.Sc. Book List            278

Thank you            281

About the author            282

# List of Illustrations

**Illustration 1:**
Repetitive arm movements in weight lifting results
in toned arm muscles                                        04

**Illustration 2:**
Untoned legs and thighs                                     04

**Illustration 3:**
Muscles must be used correctly to get the best results     05

**Illustration 4:**
Improper standing (bent knees) may result in problems
with joints and the whole body                             06

**Illustration 5:**
Various beautiful flower species created by the Creator    28

**Illustration 6:**
Various natural and beautiful gifts of love from our
Creator for us                                             29

**Illustration 7:**
Natural repair system, growth, and healing in humans      30

**Illustration 8:**
Our various bad habits causes poor body posture           31

**Illustration 9:**
Meridians throughout the whole human body
according to Chinese acupuncture                           32

**Illustration 10:**
Reflexology zones in the human body                        33

**Illustration 11:**
Reflexology points on the soles of the feet               33

**Illustration 12:**
The Healthy Eating Pyramid (Food Pyramid)          **40**

**Illustration 13:**
A plate based on the recommended balanced diet          **41**

**Illustration 14:**
Difference in the meal of someone who understands
nutrition and someone who does not          **42**

**Illustration 15:**
Body weight pressing the soles of the feet in an
incorrect manner          **43**

**Illustration 16:**
Body weight is pressing inwards or outwards          **43**

**Illustration 17:**
Stepping correctly          **44**

**Illustration 18:**
Various leg shapes          **45**

**Illustration 19:**
Distance between left foot and right foot too close
together or too far apart          **46**

**Illustration 20:**
The spine and the two hip bones as its foundation          **47**

**Illustration 21:**
Hips that are not parallel put pressure on the spine          **48**

**Illustration 22:**
Taking steps that are too wide may cause joint
and spine problems          **49**

**Illustration 23:**
Guidelines to balanced and proper walking          **50**

**Illustration 24:**
Various segments of the spine          **56**

**Illustration 25:**
Relationship between the spine and internal organs                58

**Illustration 26:**
Lungs within the chest cavity, far away from
the fingers but when the fingers are being tensed,
breathing is restricted.                                          61

**Illustration 27:**
Table (Body Systems)                                             62

**Illustration 28:**
Swinging the right leg directly to the right                     66

**Illustration 29:**
Right leg is swung to the right by first circling in front       67

**Illustration 30:**
The ideal distance between front foot and back foot:
half the foot length                                             68

**Illustration 31:**
Finding the ideal distance between left foot and
right foot                                                       70

**Illustration 32:**
Measuring the distance between the left foot and
right foot                                                       70

**Illustration 33:**
Various placements of the body weight on the sole
of the foot                                                      74

**Illustration 34:**
Various directions of the feet                                   75

**Illustration 35:**
Direction of the front knee                                      75

**Illustration 36:**
Various conditions of the knees                                  76

**Illustration 37:**
High-heeled shoes                                                    92

**Illustration 38:**
Effects of footwear with overly soft soles                          92

**Illustration 39:**
Footwear with uneven soles                                          93

**Illustration 40:**
Footwear with soles that are too thin                               93

**Illustration 41:**
Flip-Flops/thongs/sandals                                          94

**Illustration 42:**
Shoes with worn out soles                                          94

**Illustration 43:**
Placing a wallet in the back pocket                                 95

**Illustration 44:**
Carrying a bag on one shoulder                                      95

**Illustration 45:**
Hippocrates and the Hippocratic Oath                               98

**Illustration 46:**
The whole body will be more sculpted and toned                     99

**Illustration 47:**
Benefits of walking properly                                       100

**Illustration 48:**
Swinging the leg                                                   104

**Illustration 49:**
Swinging the leg outwards before forwards                          105

**Illustration 50:**
Swinging the leg inwards before forwards                           105

**Illustration 51:**
Back leg must stay relaxed     **106**

**Illustration 52:**
Back leg must continue to be directed forwards     **106**

**Illustration 53:**
Hips parallel after leg swing (proper) vs. hip pulled
forward (improper)     **107**

**Illustration 54:**
Proper front-back distance vs. a stride that is too wide     **107**

**Illustration 55:**
Body weight centered (proper) vs. body weight to
one side (improper)     **108**

**Illustration 56:**
Proper stance vs. improper stance     **108**

**Illustration 57:**
Natural healing with SONW     **116**

**Illustration 58:**
SONW reverses the ageing process because of the
improper use of the body     **117**

**Illustration 59:**
General parts of the legs and feet     **120**

**Illustration 60:**
Distance and alignment of the left foot and right foot     **120**

**Illustration 61:**
How to place the sole of the foot on the ground     **122**

**Illustration 62:**
Sole of the foot stepping evenly on the ground     **122**

**Illustration 63:**
Walking straight (proper) and not walking
straight (improper)     **123**

**Illustration 64:**
Keys 1-6 SONW                                          126

**Illustration 65:**
The use of keys in SONW                                127

**Illustration 66:**
Key 1: Swinging the Leg                                130

**Illustration 67:**
Shifting of the body weight between the front foot
and back foot prior to and following Key 1:
Swinging the Leg                                       131

**Illustration 68:**
Shifting of the body weight between the left foot and
right foot prior to and following Key 1: Swinging
the Leg                                                131

**Illustration 69:**
Left and right hips not parallel                       132

**Illustration 70:**
Knees not relaxed resulting in them being locked       133

**Illustration 71:**
Sole of the foot too close to the ground               133

**Illustration 72:**
Distance between the front foot and back foot too close  134

**Illustration 73:**
Distance between front foot and back foot too far      134

**Illustration 74:**
Stomping the heel                                      135

**Illustration 75:**
Body weight is placed too much on the front leg       135

**Illustration 76:**
Pulling the front leg down                                       136

**Illustration 77:**
Lifting the knees too high                                       136

**Illustration 78:**
Key 2: Pumping the Pad of the Foot                              140

**Illustration 79:**
Shifting of the body weight between the front foot
and back foot before and after Key 2: Pumping the
Pad of the Foot                                                 141

**Illustration 80:**
Shifting of the body weight between the left foot and
right foot before and after Key 2: Pumping the Pad
of the Foot                                                     141

**Illustration 81:**
Body brought forward at the same time as the
sole of the foot                                               142

**Illustration 82:**
The body is too far forward                                     143

**Illustration 83:**
Slamming the pad of the foot                                    143

**Illustration 84:**
Pumping with the whole leg                                      144

**Illustration 85:**
Left and right hips not parallel                                144

**Illustration 86:**
Swaying the hips when pumping the pad of the foot              145

**Illustration 87:**
Only the pad of the foot pressing on the ground               145

**Illustration 88:**
Knees not directed straight forward                                    **146**

**Illustration 89:**
Thighs not directed straight forward                                   **146**

**Illustration 90:**
Front foot turning outward/opens too wide                             **147**

**Illustration 91:**
Back foot turning outward/opens too wide                              **147**

**Illustration 92:**
Key 3: Gliding the Body While Rolling the Back Foot          **150**

**Illustration 93:**
Shifting of the body weight between the front foot
and back foot before and after Key 3: Gliding the Body
While Rolling the Back Foot                                            **151**

**Illustration 94:**
Shifting of the body weight between the left foot and
right foot before and after Key 3: Gliding the Body
While Rolling the Back Foot                                            **151**

**Illustration 95:**
Back leg and back foot are pushed: pelvis of the
back leg receives pressure, and the back leg will
be too dominant                                                        **152**

**Illustration 96:**
Body is too far forward beyond the front foot               **152**

**Illustration 97:**
Back leg not supporting the body                                       **153**

**Illustration 98:**
Looking downwards                                                      **153**

**Illustration 99:**
Body weight not evenly spread over the sole of the foot   **154**

**Illustration 100:**
Key 4: Letting All Adjustments Happen                155

**Illustration 101:**
Stomach pushed out or protruding forward            158

**Illustration 102:**
Adjusting the spine or body on your own             158

**Illustration 103:**
Lazy part of the body (knees)                      159

**Illustration 104:**
Key 5: Letting Go of the Body Weight Into the Earth   162

**Illustration 105:**
Body weight not released into the earth            163

**Illustration 106:**
Body weight released to the side                   163

**Illustration 107:**
Swinging the back leg forward                      166

**Illustration 108:**
Shifting of the body weight between the front foot and
back foot before and after Key 6: The Next Step    166

**Illustration 109:**
Shifting of body weight between the left foot and
right foot before and after Key 6: The Next Step   167

**Illustration 110:**
Dragging the back foot forward                     167

**Illustration 111:**
Curving the foot outwards                          167

**Illustration 112:**
Curving the foot inward                            167

**Illustration 113:**
The improper way of climbing up the stairs                    **180**

**Illustration 114:**
The proper way of climbing up the stairs                      **180**

**Illustration 115:**
The improper way of climbing down the stairs:
back knee is not bent                                         **181**

**Illustration 116:**
The proper way to climbing down the stairs: bend the
back knee before bringing down the front foot to land
on the pad, followed by the heel                             **181**

**Illustration 117:**
SONW workshop in Jakarta, Indonesia                          **188**

**Illustration 118:**
SONW workshop in Medan, Indonesia                            **188**

**Illustration 119:**
SONW workshop in Bandung, Indonesia                          **189**

**Illustration 120:**
SONW workshop in Asheville, United States                    **189**

**Illustration 121:**
SONW workshop in Hobart, Australia                           **190**

**Illustration 122:**
SONW workshop in Hong Kong                                   **190**

**Illustration 123:**
Before and after Pat (neck and posture improvement)          **197**

**Illustration 124a:**
Before and after Wung Hun Moi                                **200**

**Illustration 124b:**
Before and after Wung Hun Moi                    200

**Illustration 125:**
Before and after Agnes                           202

**Illustration 126:**
Before and after Gia's alopecia improvement      216

**Illustration 127:**
SONW Center Jakarta, Ketapang                    221

**Illustration 128:**
SONW Center Ivory Hotel, Bandung                 222

**Illustration 129:**
SONW Center BPH, Bali                            222

**Illustration 130:**
Elderly practicing at SONW Center                223

**Illustration 131:**
SONW Center, South Jakarta                       223

**Illustration 132:**
SONW Center, South Jakarta                       224

**Illustration 133:**
SONW Center, Asheville, United States            224

# List of Experiments

**Experiment 1:**
Recognising the connection between the way          08
we walk and negative emotions

**Experiment 2:**
Pressing the inner or outer part of the soles of the feet    42

**Experiment 3:**
Distance between left foot and right foot too close
together or too far apart                            45

**Experiment 4:**
Walking without swinging the legs                    47

**Experiment 5:**
Distance between the front foot and back foot too wide    48

**Experiment 6:**
Listening to your body through your breathing        59

**Experiment 7:**
The way we swing our legs produce different results    66

**Experiment 8:**
Swinging one leg forward                             103

# Preface

"How properly do you walk?"

"Do you consider your walk a good quality healthy walk?"

These two questions may sound strange to us. We may have heard quite often that walking can improve one's health and how there is a difference between walking in a polluted area vs. walking in fresh air, or that a 10-minute walk is not enough/that we should walk for at least 30 minutes daily. However, not too many people have thorough discussions about whether a walk is already proper or whether a walk is low-quality or high-quality. These two questions regarding the way we walk and how properly we walk is for the sake of our health.

The way we walk affects our health: improper walking harms our health; proper walking improves our health. Some of us may have heard directly from older people who said that they have knee or back problems. These conditions have become so common that we accept them as a part of getting older. However, the truth is, as soon as we fix the way we walk, the hips, thighs, and legs become toned, and the pain and aches can disappear. Some people who had already been diagnosed by doctors with such serious problems that the only option was to get surgeries ended up reclaiming their health after walking properly. I have also met 60, 70-year olds whose knee, waist, hip, and back problems disappeared after practicing high-quality walking.

From this book, you will be able to evaluate your own walk

to tell whether you have "a high-quality walk"/ "a healthy walk" or not. This book presents specific details on improper walking and its damaging effects on the body: you will discover the wrong way of walking and some of the causes. It is important to know that a prolonged improper walk not only hurts our joints and bones but also affects the spine, which is very much related to the health of our vital organs. The great news is: proper walking fixes and cancels out the problems caused by improper walking, and proper walking works not only on superficial level such as the shape of your body but also on your bones, joints, and organs, as well as your body's amazing self-healing capabilities. Some medical studies are presented in this book, and you can also read various testimonials from those who have experienced benefits from high-quality/proper walk.

Tips on how to walk properly and relevant information will be given so that you can understand the connection between walking and the body's repair system and healing process that may sound too good to be true but IS true because all of these are already naturally available to us. Proper and natural walking can truly give amazing results for your overall health improvement.

This book is a collection of tips from Secrets of Natural Walking® (SONW®) workshops that have helped thousands of people to say goodbye to their health problems, giving them a good quality of life, free of health complaints. If you are interested in getting maximum results, although I do present detailed information on SONW® in this book, I suggest you to take the workshop with an authorized SONW® instructor who has gone through intensive training who can give you personalized guidance. Secrets of Natural Walking® workshops are available in many cities in various countries.

I myself teach Secrets of Natural Walking® Workshops

(Level 1, Dancing SONW®, Level 2, and Level 3) all over the world, and I too practice SONW® 45 minutes to 60 minutes each day. I can attest that SONW® offers extraordinary benefits. My waistline size has decreased without having to do as many sit ups as I had to. It has been four years, and with regular SONW® practice, my waistline stays at its ideal size. My overall health and my stamina also have improved with routine Secrets of Natural Walking® practice.

I hope you can use the information on both improper walking and proper walking to benefit not only yourself but also others so that we all can be healthier, more relaxed, and be in a better mood in our daily life.

March 2016

**Irmansyah Effendi**

# Chapter 1
## Benefits of Walking Properly

Walking is not only tremendously important for our health but is also one of the simplest and cheapest form of exercise. Most people are aware of this fact and it may even be considered general knowledge. The multitude benefits of walking have compelled many people and leading organisations to undertake further detailed research. One such organisation is the American Heart Association who found that the following benefits may be obtained just by walking at least 30 minutes a day (as quoted from *www.heart.org/en/healthy-living/fitness/ walking/why-is-walking-the-most-popular-form-of-exercise (accessed July 4th 2019)*):

- Reduce your risk of serious diseases like heart disease, stroke, diabetes and cancer
- Improve your blood pressure, blood sugar and blood cholesterol levels
- Increase your energy and stamina
- Improve your mental and emotional well-being
- Boost bone strength and reduce your risk of osteoporosis
- Prevent weight gain

However, all these wonderful benefits barely scratch the surface of the actual benefits to be had from walking properly. How is this so? Because even if you were to walk in an improper manner you will still be able to obtain these benefits. Only after understanding the proper way of walking and practicing it correctly will you obtain the additional extraordinary results.

Due to the many additional benefits of walking properly, I have categorised them into four groups as follows:

1. Body and Health
2. Mind
3. Emotions
4. Heart and Mood

## THE BENEFITS OF WALKING PROPERLY EXPLAINED

As a general rule, it may be said that the benefits of walking properly will be obtained in a holistic manner. Let us explain these benefits in greater detail:

### 1. Body and Health

- Improves our body shape (more proportional, tighter and more toned);
- Improves our body posture;
- Improves blood circulation, the respiratory system and the absorption and distribution of oxygen throughout our whole body;
- Improves metabolism;
- Improves the natural healing abilities of our body;
- Improves our connection with the earth: our body weight will no longer be pressing against our feet;
- Reduces problems (joint pain, hip pain, leg pain, foot

pain and pain in other parts caused by improper walking);

- Prevents or reduces cellulite and varicose veins;
- Prevents problems caused by improper walking and improper posture;
- Promotes cell regeneration, resulting in anti-ageing effects.

## 2. Mind

- Calms our mind;
- Calms the soul and subconscious;
- Helps us to focus and concentrate better.

## 3. Emotions

- Prevents negative emotions;
- Reduces and eliminates negative emotions.

## 4. Heart and Mood

- Helps to open our heart, be freer and directed toward the Creator;
- Improves our mood in daily life.

## HOW CAN WALKING GIVE SUCH ABUNDANT BENEFITS?

Although the benefits previously listed may appear to be "too good to be true" in that some people would consider it to be somewhat exaggerated, in reality it is not. Everything I have noted above is true, although it may not seem to make sense initially. In this regard, let us look into a few of these benefits further:

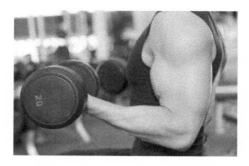

*Illustration 1: Repetitive arm movements in weight lifting results in toned arm muscles*

## 1. IMPROVES OUR BODY SHAPE (MORE PROPORTIONAL, TIGHTER AND TONED)

Looking at **Illustration 1**, if you were asked whether this person's arm will be toned if he routinely exercises by lifting weights, you will most certainly answer "yes". It is reasonable to be confident that if someone lifts weights routinely the body part involved will eventually become toned.

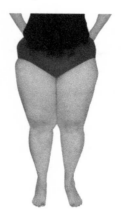

*Illustration 2: Untoned legs and thighs*

So, why would something as shown in ***Illustration 2*** below occur? In fact, why would I even ask such a question? What is the connection between how toned the arm of a weightlifter is and someone's untoned calves? You might surmise that only people who routinely exercise will have a toned body and therefore people who do not routinely exercise will have an untoned body.

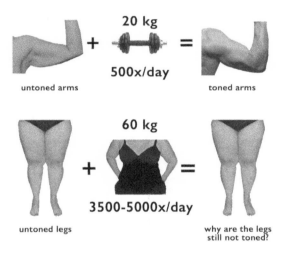

Illustration 3: Muscles must be used correctly to get the best results

Indeed, this is the most basic, most important matter for us to discuss. ***Illustration 2*** clearly shows that the person's leg and thighs are "loose" or in other words, untoned. However, aren't the thighs the part of the leg that actually supports the body? Assuming that the body weight of this person is at least 60 kilograms (kg) then each leg should support at least 30 kg each time this person is standing or walking, a substantial amount of weight. Additionally, are you aware, that according to research by Dr. Yoshiro Hatano (a professor from Kyushu University in Japan) and his team that people who seldom exercise will still walk at least around 3,500 to 5,000 steps a day? *(Source: https/www.medibank.com.au/bemagazine/post/exercise/why-you-should-walk-10000-steps-a-day)*.

Accordingly, every time a person takes a step, each of their legs will support at least 30kg, or half of his/her bodyweight. That person will walk thousands of steps each day and in general will walk each and every day.

How sure are you if the arm being used to lift a weight weighing 20kg as many as 500 times a day will become toned? Definitely, right? So, if the leg of the person in the illustration is supporting a heavier weight and is doing so much more frequently, why are the legs of many people not as toned as the arm of the weightlifter?

This is a vital issue rarely understood or realised by many people. As shown in **Illustration 3**, many people do not use their legs (including their whole body) properly. This includes the way they walk and because of that, although people in general walk at least 3,500 to 5,000 steps a day, their thighs and hips remain untoned. Actually, the body weight and the number of steps taken every day should be more than enough to tone their whole leg. This same issue also applies to the upper parts of the body such as the stomach, chest and arms.

Because the muscles in our whole body are interconnected, walking properly will not only help to tone the muscles of the whole body but also to change our body shape, not just to be more toned and/or straighter but also to be more proportional. For example, for women their breasts and buttocks will be tighter and more shaped. For men it should make for broader shoulders and more sculpted abs.

In training at the gym, you may be aware that if a particular movement is not executed correctly, the results of training will be limited and/or minimal. Conversely, if that movement is executed properly (sometimes this only involves changing the position of the arms or legs slightly), the effects on the muscles being trained are maximised. In this case, satisfactory results may be obtained in a shorter period of time.

After reading this, you may deduce that the way we stand or walk has a direct and significant effect on the health of our whole body. Our bodily organs may function much better and even illnesses afflicting our internal organs can heal. Examples of such illnesses include reduced kidney function, high levels of "bad" cholesterol and high blood sugar levels.

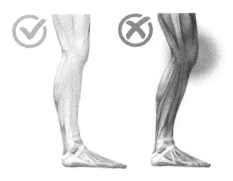

*Illustration 4: Improper standing (bent knees)*
*may result in problems with joints and the whole body*

Conversely, an improper way of standing or walking may cause problems on our joints and whole body. You may observe this issue at *Illustration 4*.

## 2. PREVENTS, REDUCES AND ELIMINATES NEGATIVE EMOTIONS

Is there a connection between our negative emotions and the way that we walk? Yes, there is, and it is indeed a close connection. Some of you who are quite sensitive may be able to feel it by conducting the following simple experiment.

### Experiment I: Recognizing the connection between the way we walk and negative emotions

Please find a spacious area that will allow you to safely take successive steps at a rapid pace.

1. Walk a few steps as if you are in a hurry and think about something unpleasant that upsets you. Be aware of the negative emotion or your reaction.

2. Walk in a relaxed manner while still thinking of the same unpleasant matter. Be aware of the negative emotion or your reaction.

If you are sensitive enough, you will be able to feel that although you were still thinking of the same unpleasant matter, while you are walking in a rush your negative emotions are much stronger compared to while you are walking in a relaxed manner. So, the way we walk certainly has a significant effect on our negative emotions. Walking in an improper manner will strengthen the existing negative emotions. Conversely, walking properly will reduce our negative emotions.

### 3. IMPROVES OUR MOOD IN DAILY LIFE

Similar to the connection between the way we walk and negative emotions, there is also a connection between the way we walk and our mood in daily life. Walking improperly will worsen our mood whilst walking properly will improve our mood.

### FOR ALL AGES

I have many friends and acquaintances who are older than 60 years who have for many years frequently complained about knee pain, hip pain, and so on. They have consulted with specialist doctors and were advised that such ailments are reasonable and natural due to their old age. They were simply suggested to exercise more often and consume glucosamine to manage their ailments. After following the recommendations of these doctors, they did feel some marginal improvements although they were often still suffering.

However, as soon as my friends corrected the way they walked, all of the ailments related to these issues disappeared completely. Lately, every time I meet them all they talk about is how their whole body had become healthier, fresher, with more stamina, their chest muscles becoming more toned and even being able to see some definition in their stomach muscles. Imagine, their days usually filled with complaints because of their aging bodies had completely changed, replaced with joy because their bodies have become heathier and fresher. Some of my friends even said that they had never felt this good, even compared to their younger days when they were still 20-30 years old. This does not seem to make sense, right? However, this is the reality as set out in their testimonials in the following section.

## SOME EXPERIENCES AFTER WALKING PROPERLY

Interestingly, correcting the way we walk is not only beneficial for older people. Young men and women who are still in their 20s and 30s have also reaped significant benefits. Note that I am not referring to people who are passive and riddled with illnesses. People who are extremely active in exercising and controlling their diet have obtained benefits that they were never able to obtain from a strict diet and intense exercise at the gym. Why is this so? A strict diet may help to lose weight, but it does not make the body more proportional. Intense exercise at the gym can improve the body shape, however for some people the changes to some parts of their body may be limited.

Also, if the gym routine is discontinued, the results tend to disappear quite quickly. Interestingly, just by improving the way we walk, we may obtain results that cannot be obtained from dieting and an intensive gym routine.

Many children, upon walking properly, have also obtained many great benefits. Those who were stressed because of academic pressure or peer pressure were able to handle their stress better, and many of them reported stress relief after proper walking. Of course, their health, energy, and emotional stability also improved automatically.

## 12-Year-Old Boy: Dyspraxia, ADHD

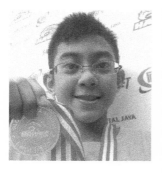

My son, Hikaru Balint Madani is a gifted child with learning difficulties. Consequently, he was moved to a special needs elementary school when he entered year 3. The learning difficulties experienced by Hikaru was diagnosed as dyspraxia, a developmental coordination disorder caused by the inability of the brain to process information. Before entering the special needs elementary school, the psychologist diagnosed Hikaru with ADHD (attention deficit hyperactive disorder) and dyslexia, a developmental disorder in the ability to read and write commonly affecting children aged 7 to 8 years. After practicing SONW level 1 for one year, Hikaru's psychologist recognised that there was a clear change in Hikaru and encouraged him to continue practicing SONW. In January 2016, Hikaru was challenged to join the SONW 21 days challenge by his friends.

Incidentally, his teammates consisted of a mum and her two boys (who lived in a different country), but they enthusiastically practiced together over Skype. Hikaru appeared to thoroughly enjoy this process together with his group. After completing the 21 days challenge, Hikaru experienced profound changes both physically and non-physically. The physical changes included:

- Becoming 2.5 cm taller;
- Gained 700 grams of body weight. This was significant to Hikaru because he had difficulties gaining weight whilst his body easily lost weight;
- 4 cm increase in chest measurement;
- 1.5 cm increase in hip measurement;
- His left and right thighs became balanced in size;
- His previously bow-legged legs became straight.

Hikaru found it difficult to gain weight although he consumed plenty and enjoyed snacking. However, after the 21 days challenge, a pleasant change occurred in his body. He found his school uniform pants to be too tight and had to loosen them. There were also changes to his bones and his shoulders were no longer sore because his body posture became straighter. Additionally, while walking day to day his legs were no longer sore and his sleep quality improved.

At school he also became more focused. His grades and scores improved, his ability to concentrate improved and stabilised, his empathy towards his classmates increased, he no longer daydreams in class, he was able to complete and submit his tasks and exams on time (previously he did not) and he was even given a reward because he was able to continuously meet targets set by his class teacher over a period of one week.

These significant changes were recognised by this therapist. But what surprised his therapist the most is that my son's ability to focus had improved significantly. This was despite missing two therapy sessions. He was considered more ready and able to actively participate in activities. Hikaru also took responsibility for his homework even though he was staying over at his grandmother's place on the weekends. Even when his cousin came over to play, Hikaru was still able to maintain his focus in completing his homework. His initiative was also exceptional. Now his ability to tell stories is excellent and structured. And what makes the least sense is the symptoms of dyslexia and ADHD had disappeared. Last year, Hikaru was able to move to International School at year 6, and already joined SONW level 3. Now he become a young artist.

This is an extraordinary gift of love from our Creator. The chance to participate in SONW and to feel the benefits is an extraordinary opportunity. As a mother, I would like to invite other parents to give your children the chance to practice SONW, especially for kids with learning difficulties. You no longer need to teach and train your kids with great difficulty to concentrate better, become more independent and think logically. SONW is good!

*Britt Hermawan, Hikaru's mother*

## 15-Year-Old Teenager: Feeling Happier and Becoming Prettier

Before I had started the natural walking I usually woke up having the mentality that I had a really long stressful day ahead of me, but once I had started the walking every morning for an hour, it re-energized me. It made me change my ways of thoughts when I looked at the day ahead. I see it now more of an opportunity to do new things rather than a long task I had to complete.

The walking has made me in general more of a cheerful and open person when it came to interacting with others. My openness has also resulted me into being more of a calm, less stressed and welcoming person which isn't only beneficial for my sake but also for the sake of my family members.

Before | After

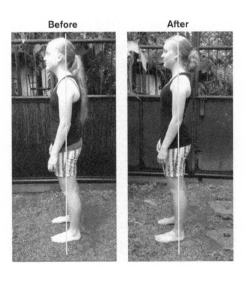

I am also more pleased when I see my reflection in the mirror: my face has cleared up from the bad skin I had; my thighs have gotten tighter; my spine holds itself upright; and my neck rests on top of my shoulders rather than it leaning too much to the front. All this has been a pleasing change, but the change that I was most delighted with was when I looked in the mirror I saw a smile that was, in my opinion, a smile I hadn't felt in a long time. It felt soft, unforced and pure. Thank you, SONW 21-Day Challenge.

*Nimue Lauritzen*

---

## 24-Year-Old Female: Improved Scoliosis, Better Body Proportions

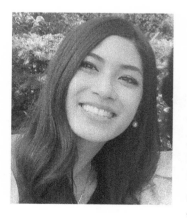

My scoliosis was mild with an 'S' shaped spine and I was diagnosed at an early age of 10. It resulted in years of discomfort. Because of the pinched nerves on my upper back, I had problems sleeping. When moving my back and shoulders, it made 'cracking' noises constantly. This got slightly worse over time and I started to accept the discomfort on my back as a part of my life.

During sports/ exercise, there were certain movements that were painful, and the doctor suggested I start practicing Pilates. I had to come in twice a week and use big machines to do simple leg lifts. After 6 months, I did not feel much difference although the exercises were supposed to strengthen the muscles around the spine to prevent further curving.

The doctors said it was impossible to straighten the spine without surgery which was only performed on serious scoliosis patients. I was also given the option of wearing a brace which would prevent the scoliosis from getting worse.

I tried not to think about not having a straight spine for the rest of my life and accepted this until SONW. I could feel my "cracking" sounds on my back decreasing. I grew an extra 2.5cm tall (1 inch) and my waist is now straight instead of curved at the spine.

*Krissan Iskandar, 24 Years Old*

---

## 54-Year-Old Male: Healthier, More Energized, More Vitality

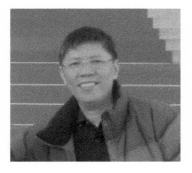

Prior to SONW, my health had never been great. In layman's terms my body was "worn out". I easily succumbed to illness such as throat inflammations, coughing fits and several other illnesses related to my digestive system. I have lived with this condition from an early age.

The first time I practiced SONW seriously and routinely was after I was infected by the chikungunya virus (similar to dengue fever). As it is well documented in relation to this particular virus, in general six months following remission, the pain will continue to persist especially in the joints. However, after routinely practicing SONW every day, my recovery post-infection was significantly more pleasant and of a shorter duration compared to what is generally experienced by others. And… without realising it, my body actually became fresher and more energised. I rarely became ill and in fact to this day I have not experienced throat inflammations and coughing fits. This is despite living in Bandung where many people were infected with such diseases. In this regard, I certainly feel that my health has improved so much that I am in better shape even compared to when I was 20 years old.

The other benefits that I did not initially recognise was the increase in my vitality, energy and libido in my intimate relationship with my wife. Evidently, by practicing SONW routinely every day, my vitality increased significantly. This is despite the general understanding that our vitality levels will decrease as we age, especially past 50 years. Notwithstanding this, after I practiced SONW, it was clear that the opposite happened. All of these benefits were obtained after practicing SONW almost every day. Since then I rarely miss a day of SONW practice.

***Darma Sukmana, Bandung, Indonesia***

## 69-Year-Old Female: More Energy, Balanced Emotions, Beautiful Body

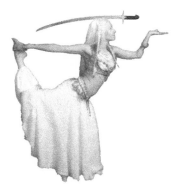

It has been two years since I first learned Secrets of Natural Walking®. Now, I can't imagine living without it. At the time I first learned SONW, I had been suffering from adrenal burnout. My ability to travel and work were limited. My required self-care, including diet, rest, calm environment, took a great deal of my time and energy. After just two weeks of practicing natural walking, I felt very different – more energized, but also calmer, more relaxed – a very important component to healing the adrenals.

What amazes me most is how the simple Natural Walking practice is like getting an inner shower, releasing stress and tension throughout my being. I am a psychologist, and I don't understand why it works, but it does. Although I am a long-time meditator and find wonderful benefit from my daily meditation and prayer, the Natural Walking practice gives me something more, seeming to lighten the hold my head has on my life, to fill and cleanse me with a deep life energy that is vibrant and also restful. In all my years of personal work, study, and physical practices, including chi gung, a life time practice of hatha yoga, dance, and outdoor sports, I have felt nothing like it. It is as if the deep rivers of the body and energy are flowing as they should, which in turn nourishes all of the physical systems of the body and mind.

One of my favourite effects of Natural Walking is the balancing of my emotions. Imagine feeling down, and just taking a few slow steps, as we do with the Natural Walking, and as you walk feeling more and more uplifted, as if an invisible hand was lifting your mood from the inside. It fascinates me. I am a researcher by training, and a sceptic by nature. Every day I am doing my own research and watching others have the same experience I am having…. of lightening, brightening, calming and becoming more energized.

Another dramatic benefit for me has been the effect on my self- imposed ageism. Before SONW, I was getting OLD. I am 69 after all, so I was allowing myself to begin the gentle winding down of the upper middle aged, coasting into retirement, life in the garden, telling myself I may as well face and enjoy a downhill ride. I cannot put my finger on what happened, it was like a switch was changed. I don't just feel younger physically, I feel very different on the inside, as if years don't have the same effect on me. My posture is more alert and alive. I am no longer looking down the hill, but at the plain, a wide-open expanse of possibilities available. Life has picked me up again and doesn't look like it is about to let me go.

And then there is my body….ah yes. Middle age sag had set in, not too badly as I was a regular yoga practitioner, a dance teacher, and loved to hike weekly up the hills around my home. But old skin just doesn't cover up things the way young skin does. I remember a moment two years ago, looking at my legs and saying to myself, "well, it's down from here. I may as well just accept it." Not a month later I was in my first SONW class. And yes, it has been up. Not that I'm ready to be a pin-up, but my man sure is happy with how I look. I've lost inches here, and toned there, and generally feel much more comfortable in my body – and that with only doing the walking practice for the last three years, as I took a hiatus from yoga and dance.

*Diana Stone, Ph.D., Psychologist, 69 Years Old*

## It Even Healed a Yoga Teacher

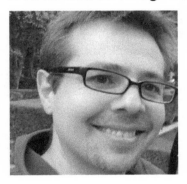

Almost two years ago I started practicing what I now believe is the most powerful, natural and effective exercise ever. I make this statement after being a long-distance runner for over 30 years, completing over 10 marathons, multiple triathlons (including 2 Ironmans), learning tai chi, practicing yoga daily for 8 years, and becoming a certified yoga teacher. So, what is this amazing new exercise? Allow me to introduce you to the Secrets of Natural Walking®. At the core of this "natural walking" is a deep realization that the body is an amazing system that if treated properly can naturally heal itself. This concept is far from new, as many people have an understanding that the body has a propensity to self-heal. For example, when you cut your finger, if you wash the cut and apply gentle pressure to stop the bleeding, the body will heal the cut, often to the point of being invisible on the skin. Yet most people don't realize the many things they do that put stress on their body systems, inhibiting the body's ability to heal

Walking is something we, as humans, do a lot of, as our primary means of mobility. The average person takes between 3,000-10,000 steps per day. This amounts to well over a million steps per year for most! Walking is a wonderful way to exercise muscles, while burning calories and getting fresh air. Many benefits of walking are already well known. However, what is not well known is that most – if not all – people put too much pressure on their joints and bones when walking, while not engaging the proper muscles. After taking thousands and thousands of steps, we slowly start to wear out the cartilage in our joints, using only some of our muscles while others atrophy away. Improper walking also puts pressure on our body organs and doesn't allow our energy meridians and reflex zones to function for proper self-healing. This actually deteriorates our bodies, making us less healthy and shortening our life spans. In order to reduce the wearing out of our joints, reduce degeneration of our muscles, and properly activate the energy meridians and reflexology zones in our bodies, we need proper alignment and balance in our step. Just as a balanced nutritional diet helps the human body thrive, proper walking is just as important. There are so many things proper walking can help with, and I am one of the thousands of people who are the walking proof of some of the wonderful 'miracles' experienced.

Since I was about 10 years old, my parents started noticing my bad posture. While I was constantly reminded to 'straighten my back' I could only do it for a few seconds, or minutes at best, before regressing to my comfortably hunched back. My spine's curvature began to worsen, so my parents tried a number of things to help, including using back braces, going to chiropractors, doing prescribed back exercises, hanging for extended periods of time on stall bars or gym ladders, etc. None of these worked, so my parents eventually gave up. At a similar age, I also got asthma, which I believe was somewhat related to my mild case of kyphosis (a type of scoliosis). I had to live with my hunched back, which not only looked unattractive but lead to some less than endearing nicknames such as "Quasimodo" or the 'Hunchback of Notre Dame'.

After college I got heavily involved in triathlons. During my training and events, my back would often hurt especially during cycling as I had to bend over the handlebars and I usually put the strain on the curved part of my back. I eventually got various mild repetitive foot injuries (mostly from running) and decided to take a break and focus on yoga to help strengthen muscles. I got very involved in yoga, taking rigorous 90 min classes daily, attending many week-long yoga retreats, eventually completed yoga teacher training certification. Yoga did many things for me including becoming more flexible, strengthening back and core muscles, and improving my balance. I was able to keep my posture straighter due to strengthening my back muscles and increasing my lower back flexibility. However, my back still was curved, and when I was tired/lazy to engage my back muscles, my posture reverted to the way it was before.

About 2 years ago I learned about the Secrets of Natural Walking® in a daylong workshop where I learned how to retrain my body to walk properly and naturally using 6 keys. Using the 6 keys, we allow the muscles in our bodies to engage naturally without forcing or tensing them. Among the many things learned at the workshop, one of my main takeaways was the incorrect way my weight was shifting while walking which encouraged my overly curved spine. About a week after I took the workshop, I already noticed my spine naturally beginning to straighten, although this was not without experiencing quite a bit of soreness in the lower/middle part of my back where my kyphosis began. I measured myself 3 weeks after the workshop and noticed between a 3/4 and 1 inch growth! After another 2 weeks I was at about 1 inch taller. Now after close to 2 years of regularly doing the exercise my spine is almost normal shape and I've gotten close to 2 inches taller! The straightening of my spine is happening all the way from my pelvic bone to my head. Additionally, I'm noticing muscles appear in my abdomen, chest and back that I've never felt before, as a result on the natural walking. Indeed, it works on practically all the major muscles in the body.

This is not the only improvement I've experienced since doing the natural walking practice. My eyesight has also improved 1.0 dioptre in each eye. My right eye previously required a lens of -2.25 and my left eye a lens of -2.0. Now I wear glasses with -1.25 in my right eye and -1.0 in my left eye. In addition, my outward rotation of my right leg has been re-aligned to normal position. My health/immune system has also improved as the frequency of me getting colds dropped from 3-5x per year to 1x per year, with the duration of cold also decreasing from 2-6 days to 1-2 days.

Incredibly, there is even more. About 3 years ago I got into a near fatal cycling accident – breaking 7 ribs, my collarbone and shoulder blade and one of my lungs partially collapsed. After a few months of healing and great recovery, my right shoulder sagged quite a bit due to muscle atrophy and the lack of bone support from the broken ribs, collarbone and shoulder blade. What happened during the natural walking practice was amazing. I could actually feel pops and clicks in my shoulder and right chest area during the natural walking exercise as the muscles there began to naturally engage to support my sagging shoulder. After the natural walking exercise my right shoulder would be noticeably higher than before that particular natural walking exercise session. I would experience these sounds and adjustments initially only when I did the natural walking exercise. Over time as my normal walking began to change and become more proper, I would also begin to feel the adjustments occasionally during normal walking as well. This further strengthens my belief in the power of natural walking.

A few months after taking my first natural walking workshop, I stopped practicing yoga. This is because I want to use my limited free time to practice natural walking as much as I can (up to 90 minutes per day if possible), as I saw significantly more benefits on my body and health from natural walking than yoga. However, while I knew that I would get the adjustment/alignment benefits as well as core and leg muscle strengthening from natural walking, I didn't realize that I would also get more flexible, which is another core aspect of yoga. With natural walking my hamstrings and lower back, which have always been abnormally tight – which I believe is related to my kyphosis, are getting more flexible. This flexibility is similar to what I experience with a complete yoga workout, but with natural walking it is less painful and more natural!

Natural walking engages pretty much every muscle in our bodies. Can walking "work-out" most muscles in your body, including the abs, chest and arms? Yes! I was surprised too but walking actually should engage the majority of our muscles in the most balanced and natural way. Now I can feel many of these upper body muscles engage when I walk naturally! We shouldn't have to perform isolated exercises with weights or machines (e.g. Circuit training) to properly exercise our muscles or getting into various yoga asanas/poses. By using our muscles in a balanced and proper way while doing something as simple/natural as walking (and sitting/standing), most body problems – including pains from joints in our knees, hips, back, shoulders and neck will naturally go away. Even pain in the elbows and wrists – carpal tunnel for example, can reduce significantly – there are numerous cases of people with these problems who noticed significantly reduction or cures with natural walking. My digestion has also improved, and whenever I have an upset stomach a few minutes of natural walking practice usually takes care of it. This exercise is also low impact – meaning there is minimal chance of injury, none if done properly. It can be done by everyone of all ages. The only requirement is that the person can walk either on their own or with an assistive device (cane, walker, etc.). This exercise doesn't require going to a special location, like a gym, fitness center, track, or even outside. It can be done in your home. As the exercise is done barefoot (more natural), it doesn't require any special equipment, like fitness clothes, sneakers/shoes or other special equipment that can end up costing tens to hundreds of dollars. Simple and natural. I encourage you to experience it for yourself by taking a one-day workshop that explains how to practice regularly this 'perfect' exercise on your own. And I'd love to hear about the health benefits you receive.

*John Benko, San Francisco, California, U.S.A.*

## Assists in Recovery of External and Internal Wounds of a Kyokushinkan Expert

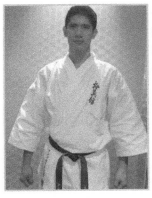

As a full-contact martial artist, I often get serious injuries from participating in tournaments, championships, and even at practice at the dojo.

In an attempt to heal external and internal wounds in training and competitions, I have tried many alternative healing methods to assist in recovery but found that they took a long period of time. This hampered my ability to perform at my peak.

However, after learning SONW, the healing of all external and internal wounds became faster. Even my stamina and strength increased significantly.

After realising how beneficial SONW is I decided to join the special training and sit the exams to become a SONW instructor to be able to share this SONW to others.

*Danny Pajouw, Brand Chief at Kyokunshinkan International Indonesia*

## Chronic Skin Spots Disappeared

I joined SONW first time in March 2014. In my profession I have a lot to do with music and movement and body consciousness. Therefore, I thought that I knew quite well how to walk properly. When joining the workshop, I realised, I did not know at all, what is proper. Since then I continuously got and get so many benefits. Among them:

- I had a really big spot in my face, a brown wart. It is nearly gone.
- I regularly had pain in the joints of my toes and fingers, especially in the morning, when starting to move. No pain anymore.
- After giving birth to three wonderful daughters, my pelvic floor muscles were damaged. With every jump, cough or sneeze I would wet my clothes. I can jump around again!
- My feet had become one size bigger after the pregnancies. My feet came back to the old size.
- Nothing used to help me, when having pain on my neck and back. Today, if pain comes up, doing the SONW diligently, takes care of all pain.

I am so grateful for this indescribable gift of SONW!

*Ursula Granitza, Germany*

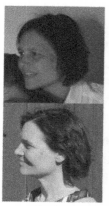 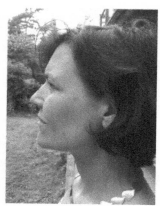

**BEFORE**          **AFTER**

# Chapter 2
## The Human Body is A
## Gift of Love from Our Creator

We often forget one basic but extremely important matter about our body. What is it? That our body is a creation of our Creator. You might say that you have not forgotten, that you and many others have always remembered that our body is a creation of our Creator. You might even ask, is this not general knowledge? Yes and no. Why do I say yes and no?

Although most people are aware that the human body is a creation of our Creator, this piece of knowledge in isolation is limited and superficial. Most people do not truly understand the real meaning of our body being a creation of the All Loving and Caring Creator. Why is this so?

Remember that we are talking about the All Loving and Caring Creator. Let us contemplate about the meaning of the words the "All Loving and Caring Creator". To illustrate, consider that compared with how much we might love our parents, siblings, or children, for sure our Creator's love for us must be even greater.

As proof, let us observe the beautiful flowers around us.

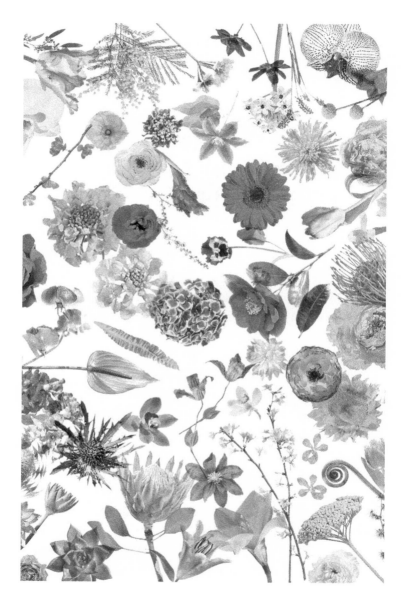

*Illustration 5: Various beautiful flower species created by the Creator*

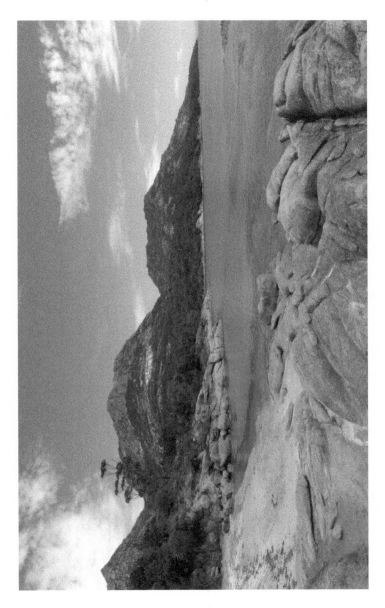

*Illustration 6: Various natural and beautiful gifts
of love from our Creator for us*

*Most people do not know the true meaning of the human body being a creation of the All Loving and Caring Creator.*

There are so many types of flowers in various colours that the our Creator has created for us *(see Illustration 5)*. Let us also examine the various trees and other plants also created by the our Creator. Other than this there is also the sky, clouds, mountains, rivers, beaches and other beautiful things around us *(see Illustration 6)*. Everything is the creation of the All Loving and Caring Creator to bring joy to us. If we realise the existence of all of this, then how beautiful should our Creator's gift to us, our body, be? It must certainly be even more beautiful than all of those other gifts.

## THE EXTRAORDINARY REPAIR, GROWTH AND NATURAL HEALING CAPABILITIES

As you are aware, if we injure our skin it will naturally heal, broken bones will also heal, and hair will also grow back. Every single day we shed millions of cells that are replaced with new cells *(see Illustration 7)*.

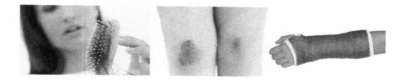

*Illustration 7: Natural repair system, growth, and healing in humans*

All of these are just a small part of the abilities that our Creator has given to our bodies. By remembering all of this, it is time for us to realise that our Creator has actually given all the best things for our body. However, it is the way we use our body in our daily life that causes many of these gifts to not function properly or even at all.

In fact, many of our daily habits impacts negatively on our body posture which causes various health problems. In this modern era, more and more gadgets make us use our body incorrectly. For example, many people use their mobile phones for hours without realising its negative effects on their body posture *(see Illustration 8)*.

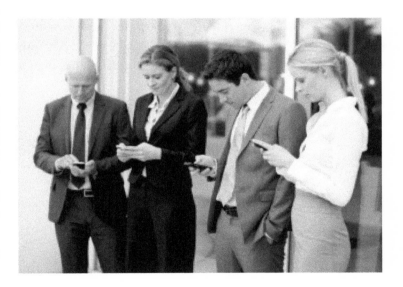

*Illustration 8: Our various bad habits causes poor body posture*

Now let us return to our previous discussion about our Creator's gift for our body. Our body was certainly granted the various means of repair, growth and healing. Apart from the ability to heal external wounds, broken bones, regrow hair loss, and the regeneration of cells that we had already discussed, let us look further into our body's ability to repair, regrow and heal itself.

You would certainty have heard about Chinese acupuncture which is a technique rooted in the basic principle that there are acupuncture points and meridians all over the body which connect the whole body together *(see Illustration 9)*. If someone is experiencing health issues, it must be because there are blockages in their meridians. Chinese acupuncture will unblock the blocked meridians to allow the body's natural healing abilities to heal the body. Thus, Chinese acupuncture does not directly heal the body but simply helps the body's natural healing process.

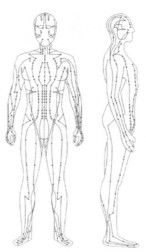

*Illustration 9: Meridians throughout the whole human body according to Chinese acupuncture*

Similar to Chinese acupuncture is the technique of reflexology. In reflexology, the human body is divided into ten vertical zones as shown in ***Illustration 10***.

The tips of these reflexology zones are located on the soles of our feet and the palms of our hands, noting however that reflexology is more commonly associated with the feet. The tips of the reflexology zones are stimulated by pressing specific points on the feet in order to activate them. This will activate the natural functions to heal problems in our body.

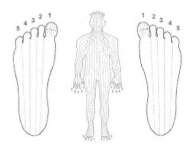

*Illustration 10: Reflexology zones in the human body*

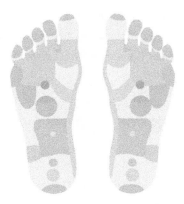

*Illustration 11: Reflexology points on the soles of the feet*

The most important matter I would like to bring to your attention is that our body inherently has numerous natural abilities to repair, grow and heal itself, but oftentimes these abilities are not allowed to function properly. We tend to block these natural abilities, even to the point that they cease to function at all. Other than that, we also tend to use our body in an incorrect manner, including walking improperly, ultimately causing diseases.

The body's natural ability to repair, grow and heal is not merely to help relieve trivial issues. Indeed, it involves many matters beyond our expectations. Problems with our muscles, bones, joints, nerves, body posture and even internal organs can all be repaired by the body's systems.

This is the meaning of realising that our body was created by our Creator. Our Creator did not only grace us with a beautiful body, but also provided the accompanying facilities to heal the myriad of problems that might afflict our body. For as long as our body functions in the most natural way, so will the facilities to heal this body of ours.

> *The aim of covering a wound is simply to prevent us from disturbing that part of the skin. A cast for a broken arm is to protect the arm from us disturbing it.*

## EVERYTHING FUNCTIONS PROPERLY WHEN NOT DISTURBED

Knowledge about the various means of reparation, growth and healing of our body is important. In this regard, let us discuss this matter and consider two simple examples that you may easily understand:

1.  Wounded skin
2.  Broken bones

## WOUNDED SKIN

If there is a part of our skin that gets wounded, but no infection occurs, what must we do to heal that wound? Of course, the wound should be cleaned thoroughly in the first instance. However, following this, usually small wounds are covered with a bandage and larger wounds are first stitched before being covered with a bandage. Although it may appear that we are doing something to heal the wound, what we have actually done is simply to cover the wound to stop us from disturbing it. The wounded skin will in time heal itself if we do not disturb it. If we were to rub and scratch the wounded skin every few minutes the wound would never heal, right?

## BROKEN BONES

The same applies for broken bones, the treatment a doctor applies is similar in principle to the case of the wounded skin. Broken bones must be protected by a cast only to prevent us from disturbing the bones. Naturally the broken bone will heal on its own (with the exception of serious cases where the bone must be replaced by a prosthetic substitute).

## IMPORTANT KEYS TO ALLOW THE BODY'S FACILITIES TO FUNCTION IN THE BEST MANNER

So, with these two examples about the healing abilities of our body, what are the key points to understand to allow the body's facilities to function as best as possible?

1.  Satisfying the body's needs
2.  Not disturbing the body

## 1. SATISFYING THE BODY'S NEEDS

In order for our body and the special facilities within to function well, we need to satisfy the body's needs, for example:

- As recommended by nutritional guidelines, we must consume nutritious food to ensure that the nutritional requirements of our body are met.

- We also need to have enough rest so that our body gets a chance to recuperate, restore, grow and heal itself.

## 2. NOT DISTURBING THE BODY

The previous two examples show that one of the most important keys to ensure that the body is able to heal itself is that we must not disturb the part of our body that is in the process of recovering.

It sounds simple, right? However, in reality, it is not as simple as it sounds. Why? Because we have been using our body improperly resulting in this bad habit sticking with our body. One of the simplest examples is poor body posture. In any condition, including when in a relaxed state, people with a poor body posture are not 100 percent normal. Poor body posture is only one example that is easily identifiable. If the structure of our body that consists of bones and joints is worn down due to our daily habits, just imagine what happens to the other parts of our body.

Notwithstanding this, all these issues may be neutralised, and the method of neutralisation is natural and can be undertaken by almost everyone. What are some natural things that most people do? These include utilising our five senses, breathing and walking. From these, walking is the one that moves the whole body. Therefore, the answer is walking. Indeed, walking is the very facility that our Creator has given us to neutralise everything that has happened because of our day to day improper attitudes and habits.

We have been using our body improperly every moment of our daily life, causing us to slow down/block/stop the natural functions of our body.

An obvious example of improper use of our body/doing something to our body/no longer letting the natural state of our body function can be seen through our body structure, expressed in our bad posture. Even when we are in a relaxed state, our posture is not 100% naturally correct. If we can't even let our major bones and joints be the way they are supposed to be, can you imagine what we are doing to the other parts of our body that are smaller and more intricate?

The great news is: the bad effects we have placed on our body can be neutralized, and the neutralization of the bad effects can be done naturally.

Walking is natural. Humans have legs, and legs are meant for walking. As a matter of fact, proper walking is the tool/the facility given to us by our Most Loving Creator to neutralize everything that we have done to our body due to our improper attitude and habits.

> *Walking is the very facility given to us by our Creator to neutralise the negative impacts of our day to day improper attitudes and habits.*

# Chapter 3
## Understanding Walking is Akin to Understanding Nutrition

Perhaps you are wondering how walking could possibly neutralise the negative effects of all our improper habits? To help you understand, let us look at the simplest daily activity we all engage in, eating. By discussing the importance of knowledge about proper nutrition for our body, you will also understand the importance of walking. Walking is not simply about moving your body from one place to another.

### GUIDELINES FOR A BALANCED DIET (FOOD PYRAMID)

You would certainly be familiar with the concept of the Food Pyramid *(Illustration 12)* which provides a guideline in preparing a healthy and balanced diet and explains that in order to meet the body's nutritional requirements, one must consume food from the various different types of food categories in the recommended amounts.

- Foundation Layer: Includes fruits, vegetables and grains making up the largest portion of the pyramid. Plant based foods contain a wide variety of nutrients like vitamins, minerals and antioxidants and are the main source of carbohydrates and fibre.

- Middle Layer: Includes dairy, legumes, fish, poultry, meat and eggs as the main source of proteins for growth and repair.
- Top Layer: Includes the healthy fats we need in small amounts to support heart health and brain function.
- Limiting alcohol, sugar, salt and saturated oils.

## THE HEALTHY EATING PYRAMID

Department of Nutrition, Harvard School of Public Health

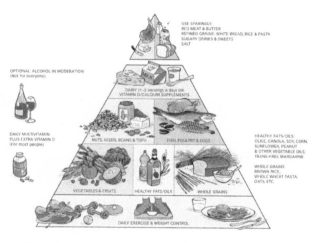

*Illustration 12: The Healthy Eating Pyramid (Food Pyramid)*

Such that our plate will resemble ***Illustration 13*** to ensure that our body is provided with the adequate amount of nutrition according to its needs.

Knowledge about proper dietary intake is so vital that many governments have implemented public policy programs to ensure that their populations are educated about healthy and proper eating. Without such education and knowledge,

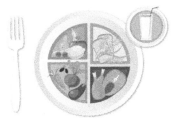

*Illustration 13: A plate based on the recommended balanced diet*

many people will only eat to simply fill their stomach without regard for nutrition or otherwise eat an unbalanced diet resulting in poor health.

Imagine if a person's diet consists exclusively of meat *(see **Illustration 14)***. Although this person will feel full, their nutritional needs will not be met because of the extreme imbalance in the diet. Further, those who are unaware of proper nutrition and health may even consume food with high sugar, salt and saturated oil content, all extremely detrimental to their health. Although one might feel full after such a diet, every time this person consumes a meal this person is also doing something harmful to their body.

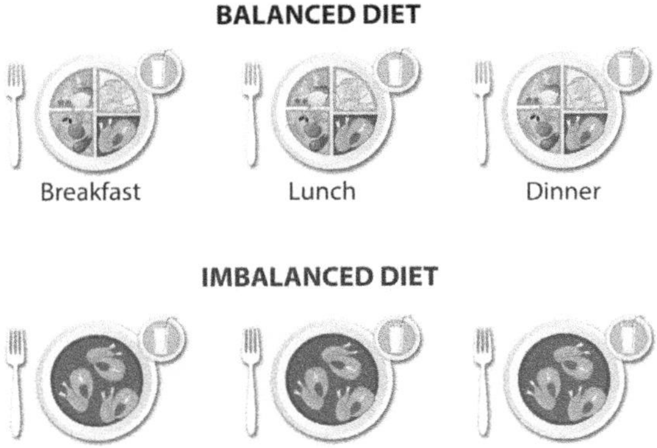

**BALANCED DIET**

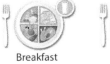  

Breakfast      Lunch      Dinner

**IMBALANCED DIET**

*Illustration 14: Difference in the meal of someone who understands nutrition and someone who does not*

If we don't understand that walking is similar in that most people consider walking simply as a means of transport from one place to another. This is similar to seeing food as only something to fill our stomach. Absent an understanding that walking is more than just a means of transport we merely move our legs without regard for anything else and indeed this is what we have been doing. What's the proof? Try the following simple *Experiments 2 to 5* and see for yourself.

### Experiment 2:
### *Pressing the inner or outer part of the soles of the feet*

In *Experiment 2*, we will examine a mistake related to improper distribution of body weight over the soles of the feet. Now try to walk the way shown in the example provided in ***Illustration 15.***

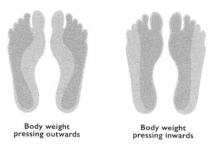

Body weight
pressing outwards

Body weight
pressing inwards

*Illustration 15: Body weight pressing the soles of the feet in an incorrect manner*

Walk six to eight steps slowly while pressing the inner part of your soles (pronation). What do you feel? Are you able to feel a tendency for your knees to press inwards when walking in this manner? If you often walk like this, the shape of your legs will eventually form the letter "X" (knocked knees) and your calves will also bend.

Conversely, if you walk while pressing the outer part of your soles (supination), your knees will start leaning outwards and in the long term the shape of your legs will form the letter "O" (bow legged). The shape of your calves will also change.

You might say that these are only experiments and in day to day life you do not walk in this manner. However, you are wrong. If you ever go to crowded places, such as the mall, take the time to observe the way people walk. Almost everybody walks in an incorrect way with many of them walking by pressing the inner or outer parts of the soles of their feet.

There are many factors that may cause a person to press the inner or outer parts of their soles while walking. One example is wearing footwear with soles that are too thick and soft. Indeed, this type of footwear is popular since it is comfortable to be worn. However, it will make your body weight easily "slide" to one side, either inwards, outwards, forwards, or backwards *(see Illustration 16)*. Whereas, your body weight should be distributed evenly over the entirety of the soles of your feet *(see Illustration 17)*. In the long term, this will affect the bone structure of your legs and your overall health.

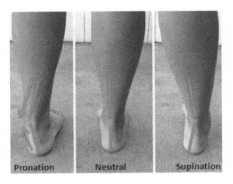

*Illustration 16: Body weight is pressing inwards or outwards*

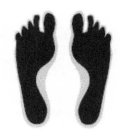

*Illustration 17: Stepping correctly*

## Notes:

There are people who are born with X or O shaped legs *(Illustration 18)*, possibly due to genetics or through contracting the Polio disease. However, a person's daily walking habits have a significant influence on the shape of their legs. Walking in an improper manner may worsen the condition and even cause deformity in legs to become X or O shaped. On the contrary, walking properly can improve the shape of our legs, so much so that the legs of a person who was born with defect or deformity, either X or O shape or other deformities may also be improved.

As seen in *Experiment 2*, if a person walks while pressing the inner or outer part of their soles, that person's legs will eventually form an X or O shape. Walking while pressing the inner or outer part of your soles is only one of the factors influencing the shape of your legs. The length, shape and various other numerous factors in each part of the legs of each person are different. In this regard, the exact shape of a person's legs may be caused by one factor or a combination of multiple factors.

In *Experiment 3*, we will observe that the distance between the left foot and right foot may contribute to the same condition. This also applies to other conditions which may be brought about by more than one cause.

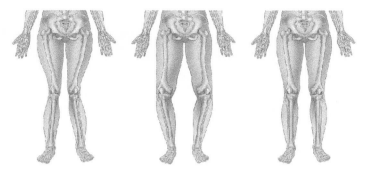

*Illustration 18: Various leg shapes*

## Experiment 3:
## Distance between left foot and right foot too close together or too far apart

Slowly walk six to eight steps maintaining a close distance between your left foot and right foot. What do you feel?

If the distance between your left foot and right foot is too close while walking, you will not step evenly (inner or outer). Depending on the shape of your legs, you will tend to press the inner or outer part of your soles, instead of evenly over the whole soles as you should.

Most people will press the outer part of their soles if their left foot and right foot are too close. However, depending on the shape, length, proportion and other parts of the person's legs, some will instead press the inner part of their soles if their left foot and right foot are too close.

Remember that a person's body weight should disperse naturally and evenly over the front, back, outer and inner parts of the soles *(see Illustration 17)*. However, this does not mean that every part of the sole should touch the ground, as the sole has a natural arch that should not touch the ground.

This is also the case should the distance between your left foot and right foot be too far apart. Depending on the shape of your legs, you will also press the inner or outer part of your soles instead of pressing evenly.

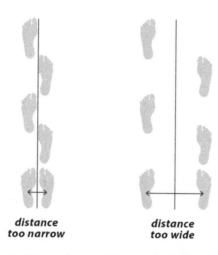

**distance too narrow**      **distance too wide**

*Illustration 19: Distance between left foot and right foot too close together or too far apart*

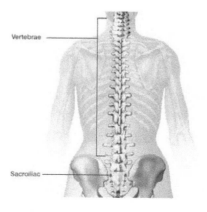

*Illustration 20: The spine and the two hip bones as its foundation*

From this experiment you are able to see how pressing the inner or outer part of the soles is something that could easily happen to many people. This habit could have started from wearing shoes with soles that were too thick and soft, or because the left foot and right foot were too far apart, and so on. These are only two examples from the many "mistakes" people make when walking.

After doing *Experiment 3* **(as shown in Illustration 19)**, you might be surprised at the number of people who make this kind of "mistake".

## Experiment 4:
## Walking without swinging the legs

Take two to four steps slowly without swinging your legs (i.e. not letting the joints of your hip work). Do this by only pushing your legs forward. What do you feel?

Are you able to feel how the hip from the side of the leg stepping forward also rotates forward, and/or that the hip from the side of the back leg also rotates until your hip is no longer parallel?

Based on **Illustration 20**, are you able to see how the left and right hips form the foundation of our spine? When the left and right hips are not parallel, or are pulled to one side, it will cause tension on the spine **(see Illustration 21)**.

Although there are flexible discs in every segment of our spine, when our hips are not parallel, there will be significant pressure placed on the spine which does not only affect our spine but will also negatively impact our whole body.

## Experiment 5:
## Distance between the front foot and the back foot too wide

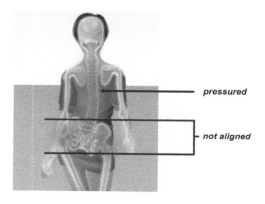

pressured

not aligned

*Illustration 21: Hips that are not parallel put pressure on the spine*

Regardless of whether your legs are swung correctly or are being pushed forward to walk, if the distance between the front foot and the back foot is too wide, the same problem as in *Experiment 4* will also happen impacting the knees, hips, and spine.

Based on these experiments, you are now able to see how easily mistakes may be made while walking. Further, the mistakes demonstrated in these experiments are only some examples of the many mistakes that someone might make while walking. These mistakes happen because we are not aware of the correct way to walk. In this regard, the way we walk is similar to the dietary choices of someone who is unaware of the concept of proper nutrition. After learning about this, do you now wish to find out more about the way you yourself walk? In **Chapter 5**, you will be invited to observe your own way of walking. By recognising the way that you walk, including the mistakes and weaknesses, I hope you will be able to correct your way of walking. By doing so, you will be able to obtain all the positive benefits of walking correctly.

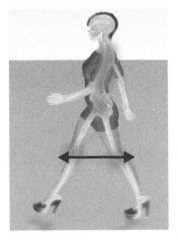

*Illustration 22: Taking steps that are too wide may cause joint and spine problems*

## THE ELEMENTS WITHIN EACH STEP

I have repeatedly mentioned that many people do not understand what it means to walk correctly, just like people eating food carelessly without regard for proper nutrition. Therefore, now let us discuss the true meaning of walking (i.e. the things that are meant to naturally happen in every step that we take). I have explained that every step is supposed to neutralise all the negative impacts from our incorrect day to day habits.

We shall now discuss the benefits of every step in further detail *(see Illustration 23)*, as follows:

- Leg muscles become tighter;
- Improvement in the condition of the bones and joints;
- Unblocking of the meridians and reflexology zones of the whole body, allowing energy to flow smoothly;
- Better posture;
- Self-healing capabilities are restored;
- Fresher and more energised, including increasing vitality;
- Improvements in the mind, emotions and mood;
- And so on.

## GUIDE TO PROPER WALKING

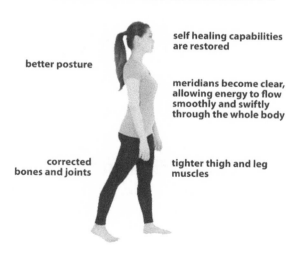

better posture

self healing capabilities are restored

meridians become clear, allowing energy to flow smoothly and swiftly through the whole body

corrected bones and joints

tighter thigh and leg muscles

*Illustration 23: Guidelines to balanced and proper walking*

By understanding nutrition, we will not eat only with the purpose to fill our stomach but will try to ensure our nutritional needs are met. Now, we also have begun to understand the real meaning of walking. Therefore, it is time for us to no longer walk simply for the sake of walking but to let the natural adjustments happen as well as possible in every step. This will not only decrease or eliminate specific health issues but will also tremendously improve our general health. Our physical posture and many other aspects will also improve on its own.

# Chapter 4
## Relationship Between the
## Way We Walk and Our Health

Following our previous discussion, is it clear that the way we walk does not only concern our "style"? At the very least we have discussed the following:

- In **Chapter 1:** walking properly can tone the legs, thighs and whole body.
- In **Chapter 2** by practicing *Experiment 2* and *Experiment 3*, you are able to see how walking improperly may result in your legs becoming X (knocked knees) or O (bow legged) shaped.
- In **Chapter 3** by practicing *Experiment 4*, you are able to see that improper walking causes pressure on the spine. As the spine is key to our health, pressure on the spine will negatively affect the whole body.

### POSTURE, SPINE AND HEALTH

Our body posture is intimately related to our spine in that a person with poor body posture will most certainly have problems with their spine. Further, a problematic spine will definitely also cause various health problems.

Based on results of recent research, the existence of a relationship between body posture and mood has been demonstrated. Try to recall a beautiful memory whilst keeping your body posture proper and straight. How do you feel? Now, hunch your body. How do you feel when your body is hunched? Repeat this experiment until you can feel the differences clearly.

Now, try to recall an unpleasant memory whilst your body posture is proper and straight. How do you feel? Now, hunch your body. How do you feel when your body is hunched? Repeat this experiment until you can feel the differences clearly.

From the above two experiments, are you able to feel a clear relationship between body posture and mood? When your body posture is proper (i.e. quite straight), your mood tends to be better. Conversely, when your body posture is improper, then your mood is also negatively affected.

## RESEARCH BY DR. ROGER SPERRY

Poor body posture is a common health issue in this modern era and is in fact much worse than many people suspect. One's posture may be said to be the "window" from which the condition of the spine could be observed. The spine has a close relationship with the brain, nerves, internal organs and organ function in general. This close relationship means that improper posture and poor spine health will directly cause a decrease in brain and organ function.

The Nobel Prize winner, Dr. Roger Sperry, stated that the spine is the motor that drives the brain. Based on his research, 90 percent of the stimulation and nutrition to the brain is generated by the movement of the spine. The remaining 10 percent of the brain's energy is utilised to process thoughts, metabolism, immunity system and healing. In this regard, Dr. Roger Sperry demonstrated that 90 percent of our brain's energy is used to process and maintain the connection between the body and gravity.

One of the worst health issues related to the spine is the disappearance of the natural arc of the spine. Ideally, we should have an arc of around 40-45 degrees in our neck, commonly referred to by chiropractors and neurosurgeon specialists as the "arc of life". This arc protects the brain stem and the spinal canal for the spinal cord and nerves that travel to every region of our body.

Subluxation is a term which describes a partial dislocation in the spine which causes pressure and irritation in the nerve channels affecting the whole body. Subluxation can cause pain but because the nerves in the spine only transmit a minimal amount of pain, many people are unaware of this issue. The loss of the arc in the neck, forward head posture and scoliosis are three types of the most dangerous types of subluxation.

*(Improvement in Forward Head Posture, Cervical Lordosis, and Pulmonary Function with Chiropractic Care, Anterior Head Weighting and Whole Body Vibration: A Retrospective Study-Mark Morningstar DC, DAASP, FRCCM, FAAIM 1, David Jockers DC, MS, CSCS2J. Paediatric, Maternal & Family Health – October 12, 2009)*

## RESEARCH BY DR. HENRY WINSOR

This following research was conducted by Dr. Henry Winsor, a medical doctor in Pennsylvania, United States of America. The University of Pennsylvania allowed Dr. Henry Winsor to conduct research into whether minor misalignments in specific areas of the spine are connected to problems with internal organs related to those areas.

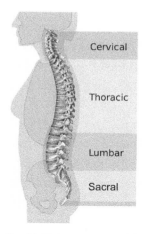

*Illustration 24: Various segments of the spine*

In three different studies, Dr. Henry Winsor undertook autopsies of 75 human bodies and 22 cats. Based on these studies, 221 parts other than the spine were found to be diseased. From all of this, 212 diseases were found to originate from the related sympathetic segment (nerve). Only in nine people it was found that the disease originated from a different sympathetic segment. Accordingly, Dr. Henry Winsor found almost a 100 percent direct correlation between minor misalignments in the spine and problems with the internal organs *(see Illustration 24 and 25)*.

**Heart Disease:**
All (20 cases) of heart disease and heart membrane with disorders exhibited misalignment of the five upper thorax segments of the spine (T1-T5).

**Lung Disease:**
All (26 cases) of lung disease exhibited misalignment in the upper spine thorax segment.

**Stomach Disease:**

All (9 cases) of stomach disease exhibited misalignment in the middle spine thorax segment (T5-T9).

**Liver Disease:**

All (13 cases) of liver disease exhibited misalignment in the middle thorax segment (T5-T9).

**Gall Bladder:**

All (5 cases) of gall bladder disease exhibited misalignment in the middle backbone thorax segment.

**Pancreas:**

All (3 cases) of pancreas disease exhibited misalignment in the middle backbone thorax segment (T5-T9).

**Spleen:**

All (11 cases) of spleen disease exhibited misalignment in the middle backbone thorax segment (T5-T9).

**Kidneys:**

All (17 cases) of kidney disease exhibited misalignment in the lower spine thorax segment (T10-T12).

**Prostate and Bladder Disease:**

All (8 cases) of prostate disease exhibited misalignment in the lower spine in the lumbar area.

**Uterus:**

Two cases of uterine disease exhibited misalignment in the second lumbar segment.

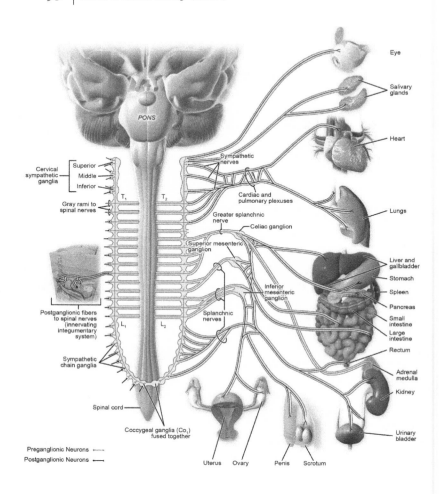

*Illustration 25: Relationship between the spine and internal organs*

This study is widely known as "The Winsor Autopsies" and the resulting report was published in November 1921 edition of The Medical Times and is available in medical libraries to this day.

*(Winsor, H. Sympathetic segmental disturbances --II. The evidences of the association, in dissected cadavers, of visceral disease with vertebral deformities of the same sympathetic segments, The Medical Times, November 1921, pp./267-271)*

These studies clearly demonstrate the relationship between our overall health and our spine. Meanwhile, the relationship between the spine and way we walk has already been discussed, for example in *Experiment 4*. Based on *Experiment 5*, it is clear that improper walking has a negative effect on the spine. Not only was the method of walking discussed in these two experiments but also the multitude of other problems which may arise from walking improperly.

## Experiment 6:
## Listening to your body through your breathing

To be able to feel the difference even more, you only need to breathe deeper without forcing yourself. Try to carry out the following experiment:

1. Stand in a proper and relaxed manner.
2. Relax and take a deep breath without forcing yourself. Feel how deep your breath is and how the muscles of your chest, stomach, etc. feel.
3. Sway your hips to one side so as to stand in a lazy manner.
4. Relax and take a deep breath without forcing yourself. Feel how deep your breath is and how the muscles of your chest, stomach, etc. feel.
5. Repeat the above steps until you can clearly feel the differences.

You can try a variation of the above experiment by replacing point 3 with just folding and tensing one of your fingers whilst still standing in a proper and relaxed manner.

Are you able to feel the differences from the above experiments? Irrespective of whether you swayed your hips or tensed your finger at point 3 of the experiment you can feel how your breath is neither as deep or smooth compared to before.

The tensing of the chest, neck and other muscles of the body puts pressure on the various organs, or otherwise does not allow them to function properly. This experiment shows how the lungs are affected merely by swaying your hips or folding and tensing one of your fingers. Because our whole body is connected, and it is clear that this pressure affects parts of our body located far from our hips or fingers, it is certain that this will also impact other organs and parts of our body.

Now try to tightly make a fist with the five fingers of one of your hands. With this action, your breathing will be affected in that it becomes shallower. At the same time, you can also feel how the muscles in your neck, chest, stomach, legs and other parts of the body also tenses up. The diaphragm, intercostal muscles, and many other muscles contributing in respiration will be more tense and limited in the movement and process.

This experiment shows and reminds us that:
- The muscles in our whole body are interconnected.
- If there is even just one part of our body being used in an improper manner, it will impact and affect many other parts of our body.

Focusing on your breathing is one of the most natural methods to understand how relaxed your body is at this current moment. Regardless of whether you are laying down, sitting down or standing for an extended period of time, your breathing will reveal your state of being. If you are unable to

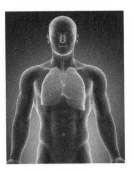

*Illustration 26: Lungs within the chest cavity, far away from the fingers but when the fingers are being tensed, breathing is restricted.*

breathe deeply, there may be parts of your body that are not relaxed enough consequently affecting the whole body.

Even if you agree with everything we have discussed up to this point, perhaps you are wondering, how would it be possible for a person to walk without any part of that person's legs or body tensing? Surely in the act of walking there will be some part of the leg or body that tenses up? There is some truth to this. For most people, there will indeed be a part of their leg or body that tenses up whilst walking, even if it is only during the course of taking one step.

You can prove this through your breathing, as has been discussed in *Experiment 6*. If you have fully understood the correct, most natural way of walking, your whole body will become more relaxed compared to when you are standing in the most relaxed way possible.

> *If you have fully understood the correct, most natural way of walking, your whole body will become more relaxed compared to when you are standing in the most relaxed way possible.*

| | Skeletal System | Muscle System | Digestive System | Respiratory System | Blood Circulation System | Urinary System | Nerve System |
|---|---|---|---|---|---|---|---|
| **Skeletal System** | | Gives something for the skeletal muscle to pull on to produce movement. | Protects the mouth, oesophagus, stomach, liver, pancreas and gall bladder. | Protects the throat, vocal chords and diaphragm. | Protects the heart. Bone marrow produces red blood cells. | Protects the kidneys. | Protects the brain and spinal cord |
| **Muscle System** | Skeletal muscles move bones. Tendons connect muscles to bone. | | Smooth muscle is found in the oesophagus, stomach, small intestines, large intestines and rectum. | The diaphragm consists of smooth muscle. | The heart consists of cardiac muscle. Smooth muscle is found in the arteries and veins. | The bladder consists of smooth muscle. | Provides protection to the nerves from the brain to the body. |
| **Digestive System** | Provides nutrition for the growth and repair of bones. | Provides nutrients for muscles to do work whether it is skeletal, smooth or cardiac muscle | | Provides nutrition for the diaphragm to allow breathing function. Important in the breathing process to generate energy. | Provides nutrition for the cardiac muscles to allow the heart to continue beating. | Provides nutrition to the kidneys so they may function to filter the blood from all toxins and residual waste from the other bodily systems. | Provides energy for the brain to allow it to process information and control all the bodily systems. |

*Illustration 27: Table: Body Systems*

|  | Skeletal System | Muscular System | Digestive System | Respiratory System | Circulatory System | Urinary System | Nervous System |
|---|---|---|---|---|---|---|---|
| Respiratory System | Provides oxygen so bones can go and do work<br><br>Removes carbon dioxide and water that skeleton cells produce as a waste product | Provides oxygen so muscles (skeletal, smooth and cardiac) can go and do work<br><br>Removes carbon waste products from the cells | Provides oxygen to the digestive system to digest food<br><br>Removes carbon waste products from the cells<br><br>Is the other half of the energy formula |  | Provides the oxygen that is carries by red blood cells to all parts of the body<br><br>Removes carbon dioxide and water that heart cells produce as a waste product | Provides oxygen so urinary system can clean the blood of waste products<br><br>Removes carbon dioxide and water that the urinary systems produces as a waste product | Provides oxygen for the brain to think and control all the other systems of the body<br><br>Removes carbon dioxide and water that the brain cells produce as waste products |
| Circulatory System | Moves oxygen and glucose around the body so cells can do the work<br><br>Moves wastes so they can be disposed by the body | Moves oxygen and glucose around the body so cells can do the work<br><br>Moves wastes so they can be disposed by the body | Moves oxygen and glucose around the body so cells can do the work<br><br>Moves wastes so they can be disposed by the body | Moves oxygen and glucose around the body so cells can do the work<br><br>Moves wastes so they can be disposed by the body |  | Moves oxygen and glucose around the body so cells can do the work<br><br>Moves wastes so they can be disposed by the body | Moves oxygen and glucose around the body so cells can do the work<br><br>Moves wastes so they can be disposed by the body |
| Urinary System | Cleans the blood of waste products by the skeletal system | Cleans the blood of waste products by the skeletal system | Cleans the blood of waste products by the skeletal system | Cleans the blood of waste products by the skeletal system | Cleans the blood of waste products by the skeletal system |  | Cleans the blood of waste products by the skeletal system |

## ALL SYSTEMS WITHIN THE HUMAN BODY ARE INTERCONNECTED

Every system within our body is interconnected and depends upon one another. For example, our skeleton system relies upon the digestive system to allow it to grow and become stronger. In the meantime, the muscle system requires the respiratory and blood circulation systems to be able to receive energy in the form of oxygen and nutrition. All these systems are required by our body to grow and develop *(www.uen.org/themepark/systems/human.shtml)*.

In light of this it is clear how body posture, spine, muscles in the whole body, internal organs and the wellbeing of the body as a whole is so interconnected. Improper walking technique will negatively impact the muscles and whole body. The most important issue to be realised however is that walking properly can repair all problems related to our posture, spine, muscles and even our organs. Simultaneously, you are also eliminating the root cause of many problems which originated though poor body posture and/or an improper way of walking.

# Chapter 5
## Common Mistakes in Walking

After gaining an understanding of how the way we walk has a significant impact on the health of our whole body, let us recognise and evaluate the way we walk in our daily lives. In this evaluation, I have attempted to include as many factors to be evaluated as possible, however each person has different habits and ways of walking. In this regard, there may be some walking habits not covered in this evaluation.

### EVEN THE WAY WE MOVE OUR LEGS MATTERS
Investigating the topic of how to walk is tremendously interesting and deep. To be able to recognise and evaluate the way we currently walk, we must undertake the evaluation based on four groups:

1. Stopping mid-walk, with the left leg in front
2. Stopping mid-walk, with the right leg in front
3. The way we swing the left leg
4. The way we swing the right leg

We must evaluate each leg separately because the way each leg steps will be different for each person. Apart from this, it is insufficient to simply undertake the evaluation after the step has been completed. The process involved in the movement of the leg must also be evaluated. To allow you to better understand, please carry out the following experiment.

### Experiment 7:
### The way we swing our legs produces different results

1. Stand with your right foot and left foot in a parallel manner.
2. Swing your right leg to step out directly to the right with a distance of approximately 50 cm from the left leg. Ensure your foot arrives solidly on the ground *(see Illustration 28)*.

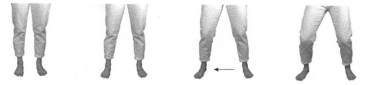

*Illustration 28: Swinging the right leg directly to the right*

3. Pat your right leg several times or ask someone to push against your right leg to feel how sturdy your right leg is. Remember to ensure your right leg is positioned solidly on the ground.
4. Stand with your right foot and left foot parallel exactly the same as in point 1, in the exact same spot (i.e. revert to the starting position).
5. Swing your right leg again to bring the sole of your right foot exactly to the same spot as in point 2 above. However, this time do not swing your right leg directly

to the right but instead bring it to circle in front of you first *(see Illustration 29).*

Are you able to feel that your right leg, following the second swinging motion, is sturdier compared to the first swinging motion? This fact is widely known by martial artists.

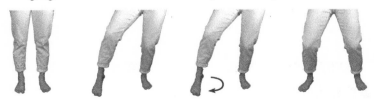

*Illustration 29: Right leg is swung to the right by first circling in front*

To ensure their "stance" is solid, they must perform a movement similar to point 5.

Although the position of the sole of the left foot and right foot, distance and so on ends up being the exact same in both the first and second movement, the sturdiness of the right leg from the second movement is vastly improved compared to the first. This has happened because in the second movement you brought your leg circling in front first before bringing it to the right. This rotation to the front causes the condition of the muscles and the muscle fibres to change compared to the first movement. So, although it may appear to be exactly the same, what occurred within the body was not the same.

Because of this, in order to evaluate the best way to walk, other than having to pay attention to each leg after each step, we also have to recognise the process within the movement of each leg.

## FINDING YOUR IDEAL DISTANCES

The shape, length and size of the various parts of our legs are different. Accordingly, a general benchmark relatively suitable for everybody must be provided. For ease and consistency, the measurements to be used will reference the size of other parts of your own body. From my experience observing thousands of people, the ideal measurements that you will obtain using this method is quite suitable for most people. Only those people with significant abnormalities should not use the following method to find their ideal distances.

## 1. DISTANCE BETWEEN FRONT FOOT AND BACK FOOT

The ideal distance between the front foot and the back foot when walking normally is ½ of the length of the sole of your foot, shown as ½ L. For clarity, see *Illustration 30*.

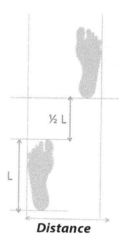

*Illustration 30: The ideal distance between front foot and back foot: half of foot length*

*Note: Should one of your feet be irregular/deformed/abnormal, please use the length of the sole of the normal foot as the benchmark.*

Measure the length of the normal sole of your foot. Write down the length of the sole of that foot in the space provided (A). Then calculate the ideal distance between the front and back foot, being (A)/2. Write down the answer as (B).

| Length of your foot | (A) _____ cm |
|---|---|
| Ideal distance between front foot and back foot<br>(B) = (A)/2 | (B) _____ cm |

## 2. DISTANCE BETWEEN LEFT FOOT AND RIGHT FOOT

The ideal distance between the left foot and right foot is exactly the width of your hip bone (not your hip). For clarity, see *Illustration 31*.

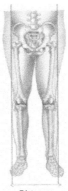

Distance

*Illustration 31: Finding the ideal distance between left foot and right foot*

Standing with your left foot and right foot as wide as your hip bone, measure the distance between your left foot and right foot in accordance with *Illustration 32.*

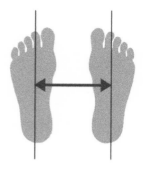

*Illustration 32: Measuring the distance between the left foot and right foot*

Write down the distance between your feet in the space provided below.

| | |
|---|---|
| Ideal distance between your left foot and right foot | _____ cm |

## INSTRUCTIONS TO EVALUATE YOUR RIGHT FOOT

Please take the time to first read the instructions outlined in this section. You do not need to memorise every single instruction, but it is simply to help you obtain an understanding in completing the table. It will be easier if someone is available to assist you to read out the instructions and write down the results of the measurements. However, even without another person's assistance you will still be able to complete this evaluation.

Then, do the following:

1. Find a place or space sufficiently spacious to carry out this evaluation.

2. Prepare a ruler or tape measure, some paper and writing instrument. You may even note down your measurements directly in the space provided in this book.

3. Without observing your legs, the way you walk, or even the way that you take each step, walk a few steps as you usually do. Stop when your right leg happens to be in front.

4. Now look at your feet and fill the Table of Walking Measurements – Right Leg (page 81) points 1 to 23. Use the "ideal measurements" as comparison.

5. Finish filling out the appropriate points.

6. Sum up your points and review the results of your walking evaluation.

## WHEN STEPPING WITH YOUR RIGHT FOOT

Walk a few more steps until you feel like you are walking as you usually do. Now, every time you finish stepping forward with your right foot, fill the **Table of Walking Measurements – Right Foot** for your right foot. Use the **Table of Walking Measurements – Left Foot** for your left foot.

## 1. DISTANCE BETWEEN FRONT FOOT AND BACK FOOT

Measure the actual distance between your front foot and back foot and deduct it by the ideal distance between your front foot and back foot. This number will be used in calculating **"finding your ideal measurement"**. Divide this difference by the ideal distance between your front foot and back foot to obtain a percentage measurement of the difference. Write down the percentage difference (E) in the table of walking measurements.

| | |
|---|---|
| Actual distance between your front foot and back foot (from measurements taken after walking as you usually do) | (C) _____cm |
| Ideal distance between your front foot and back foot (from the previous measurement) | (B) _____cm |
| Difference between actual distance and ideal distance<br>(D) = (C) – (B) | (D) _____cm |
| Percentage difference<br>(E) = (D) / (B)*100 | (E) _____% |

In relation to the distance between the front foot and the back foot, if the distance is smaller than it should be, there should be no problem in relation to the spine and body. If the difference is marginally larger than it should be it should still be no problem. However, if the distance is too large, usually the hips are no longer parallel, and the spine will be depressed.

- If E ≤ 10% whether negative or positive, mark the box "**OK**".
- If E is negative, > 10%, mark the box "**Insufficient**".
- If E is positive, >10% and ≤50%, mark the box "**Slight**".
- If E is positive, > 50% and ≤ 100%, mark the box "**Large**".
- If E is positive and > 100% mark the box "**Excessive**".

## 2. DISTANCE BETWEEN LEFT FOOT AND RIGHT FOOT

Measure the actual distance between your left foot and right foot. Ensure the part you are measuring is the same as when you were measuring the ideal distance in **"finding your ideal distance"**. Find the difference between the actual distance and ideal distance. Now, divide the difference by the ideal distance to obtain the percentage difference. Write down the percentage difference (N) in the Table of Walking Measurements.

| | |
|---|---|
| Ideal distance between your left foot and right foot | (K) _____cm |
| Actual distance between your left foot and right foot | (L) _____cm |
| Difference between your actual and ideal distance<br>(M) = (L) − (K) | (M) _____cm |
| Percentage difference in distance divided by the ideal distance.<br>(N) = (M) / (K)*100 | (N) _____% |

In relation to the distance between the left foot and right foot, whether too close or too far from the ideal distance, the consequences are both harmful. Accordingly, whether N = negative or positive is irrelevant and we will simply consider the absolute percentage figure.

- If E ≤ 10%, mark the box **"OK"**.
- If E > 10% but ≤25%, mark the box **"Slight"**.
- If not, mark the box **"Large"**.

## 3. ALIGNMENT BETWEEN LEFT AND RIGHT HIPS

Pay attention to your left and right hips. Are your hips aligned left-right, front-back and above-below?

- If everything is aligned and parallel, mark the box **"OK"**.
- If not, mark the box **"Not Aligned"**.

## 4. PART OF THE SOLE OF THE FRONT FOOT STEPPING ON THE GROUND

As discussed previously, our body weight whilst stepping might be concentrated on a particular point on the sole of the foot, when it should ideally be distributed evenly over the whole sole *(see Illustration 33)*.

For each of your feet, recognise the part of the sole that steps on the ground.

- If you are stepping properly, mark the box **"OK"**.
- If not, mark the box **"Other"** and note down the actual condition, for example **"Stepping with the outer part of the sole"**.

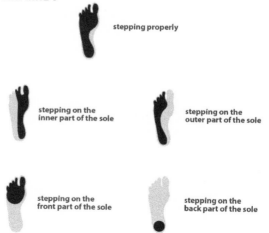

*Illustration 33: Various placements of the body weight on the sole of the foot*

## 5. DIRECTION OF THE FRONT FOOT

For each of your feet, recognise the direction of your feet in accordance with **Illustration 34.**

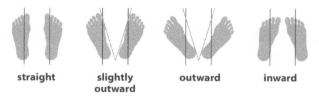

| straight | slightly outward | outward | inward |

*Illustration 34: Various directions of the feet*

- If they are directed straight forward, mark the box **"OK"**.
- If not, mark the box **"Inward"** or **"Outward"** in accordance with the actual condition.

## 6. DIRECTION OF THE KNEE OF THE FRONT LEG

For each of your legs, recognise the direction of your knees in accordance with **Illustration 35.**

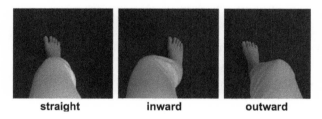

| straight | inward | outward |

*Illustration 35: Direction of the front knee*

- If directed straight forward, mark the box **"OK"**.
- If not, mark the box **"Inwards"** or **"Outwards"** in accordance with the actual condition.

## 7. CONDITION OF THE KNEE OF THE FRONT LEG

For each of your legs, recognise the condition of your knee in accordance with **Illustration 36.**

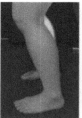 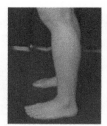 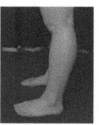

**bent knees**      **relaxed knees**      **locked knees**

*Illustration 36: Various conditions of the knees*

- If directed straight forward, mark the box **"OK"**.
- If bent, mark the box **"Bent"**.
- If locked, mark the box **"Locked"**.

## 8. CONDITION OF THE HIP OF THE FRONT LEG

For each side of the hips in relation to the front leg and back leg, recognise whether your hips are:

- Swayed to one side or straight/correct without being forced.
- If directed straight forward, mark the box **"OK"**.
- If not, mark the box **"Swayed"** or **"Lazy"** in accordance with the actual condition.

## 9. PART OF THE SOLE OF THE BACK FOOT STEPPING ON THE GROUND

Please refer to the commentary provided in **point 4**.

## 10. DIRECTION OF THE BACK LEG

Please refer to the commentary provided in **point 5**.

## 11. DIRECTION OF THE KNEE OF THE BACK LEG

Please refer to the commentary provided in **point 6**.

## 12. CONDITION OF THE KNEE OF THE BACK LEG

Please refer to the commentary provided in **point 7**.

## 13. CONDITION OF THE HIP OF THE BACK LEG

Please refer to the commentary provided in **point 8**.

## 14. WAIST AND HIP OF THE BACK LEG

Pay attention to the waist and hip of the back leg.

- If there is no pressure or any tense parts, mark the box "**OK**".
- If there is pressure on the waist or hip of the back leg, mark the box "**Pressure**".

## 15. DIRECTION OF THE BODY

Pay attention to the direction of your body (it should be directed straight forward). However, it is common for our body to be directed to the left or to the right.

- If directed straight forward, mark the box "**OK**".
- If not, mark the box "**To the Left**" or "**To the Right**" in accordance with the actual condition.

## 16. BODY POSTURE: CHEST AND BACK

Pay attention to your body posture, in particular the chest and back. The shape should be straight without being forced. However, some people's chest may be folded because their body posture is hunched.

- If naturally straight, mark the box "**OK**".
- If tense, mark the box "**Tense**".
- If hunched, mark the box "**Hunched**".

## 17. BODY POSTURE: SHOULDERS, NECK AND HEAD

Pay attention to your body posture, in particular the shoulders, neck and head. Just like the chest, the shoulders, neck and head should be straight without being forced. However, many people's necks tend to be bent downwards.

- If naturally straight, mark the box **"OK"**.
- If tense, mark the box **"Tense"**.
- If hunched, mark the box **"Bent"**.

## 18. BODY WEIGHT SHOULD BE IN THE MIDDLE

The body weight should be in the middle between the left and right legs. This allows the spine to be naturally in the middle. However, frequently our body weight tends to remain on only one leg. In this case, this produces pressure and will bend our spine.

- If the body weight is in the middle, mark the box **"OK"**.
- If not:
  - If slightly to the left or right, but not completely on either left or right leg, mark the box **"Slightly"**.
  - If completely on the left or right leg, mark the box **"On One Leg"**.
  - If swayed so much that the midpoint of the body's weight is on the outer part of one of the legs, mark the box **"Extremely Swayed"**.

## 19. FRONT LEG WHEN SWUNG FORWARD

When stepping forward, the leg should:

- Be swung properly (i.e. not being pushed).
- Not be dragged.
- Knees not being raised too high.
- Sole of the foot not being pulled downwards but being

lowered naturally.

- If the front leg is swung properly in accordance with the above description, mark the box **"OK"**.
- If not, mark the box **"Other"** and note the actual condition, for example **"Dragged"**.

## 20. FRONT LEG DIRECTLY STRAIGHT FORWARD WITHOUT ROTATING

When stepping or swinging the leg forward, the leg should be directed straight forward, not rotating inwards or outwards first.

- If the front leg is swung directly straight forward, mark the box **"OK"**.
- If the front leg is rotated inwards first, mark the box **"Inwards"**.
- If the front leg is rotated outwards first, mark the box **"Outwards"**.

## 21. SOLE OF THE FRONT FOOT WHEN STEPPING

When stepping, the heel should be placed down first, followed by the pad of the foot.

- If the foot is being placed in accordance with the description above, mark the box **"OK"**.
- If not, mark the box **"Other"** and note the actual condition.

## 22. BODY WEIGHT AS THE FRONT FOOT STEPS

Related to the method of stepping with the front foot, not only should the heel be placed first on the ground, but the weight of the leg should also be supported by the sole of the foot. After the pad of the foot has been lowered to step on the ground, the body weight will then shift downwards to be supported by the whole sole of the foot. If the body weight reaches the ground at the same time the sole of the foot touches the ground (i.e. simultaneously in one movement), it will cause you to shake. However, the worst is if the whole body weight is supported only by the heel when stepping. This will cause the heel to jerk and the consequences can be felt all the way to the spine. If the whole leg reaches the ground together with the body weight, the whole leg will shake and cause the calves to expand.

- If the heel is placed on the ground first and is only supporting the weight of the leg, mark the box **"OK"**.
- If not, mark the box **"Other"**, and note the actual condition.

## 23. BACK FOOT AS THE FRONT LEG IS SWUNG

When the front leg is being swung forward, the back leg should be relaxed, so that the back hip is not locked.

- If the step is taken as described above, mark the box **"OK"**.
- If not, mark the box **"Not Relaxed"**.

## GUIDELINES TO EVALUATE THE LEFT LEG

How we use our left and right legs in walking will usually not be exactly the same. Because of this, for the best results you are asked to repeat the same measurements on your other leg.

## TABLE OF WALKING MEASUREMENTS – RIGHT LEG

| No | Description | Results of Observation | Possible Score | Your Score |
|----|-------------|------------------------|----------------|------------|
| 1 | Distance between front foot and back foot | [ ] OK<br>[ ] INSUFFICIENT<br>[ ] SLIGHT<br>[ ] LARGE<br>[ ] EXCESSIVE | 2500<br>1000<br>1000<br>250<br>0 | |
| 2 | Distance between left foot and right foot | [ ] OK<br>[ ] SLIGHT<br>[ ] LARGE | 2500<br>1000<br>0 | |
| 3 | Alignment between left and right hips | [ ] OK<br>[ ] NOT ALIGNED | 5000<br>0 | |
| 4 | Part of the sole of the front foot stepping on the ground | [ ] OK<br>[ ] OTHER<br>_____ | 200<br>0 | |
| 5 | Direction of the front leg | [ ] OK<br>[ ] INWARDS<br>[ ] OUTWARDS | 100<br>0<br>0 | |
| 6 | Direction of the knee of the front leg | [ ] OK<br>[ ] INWARDS<br>[ ] OUTWARDS | 250<br>0<br>0 | |

| No | Description | Results of Observation | Possible Score | Your Score |
|----|-------------|------------------------|----------------|------------|
| 7 | Condition of the knee of the front leg | [ ] OK<br>[ ] BENT<br>[ ] LOCKED | 400<br>200<br>0 | |
| 8 | Condition of the hip of the front leg | [ ] OK<br>[ ] LAZY<br>[ ] SWAYED | 200<br>100<br>0 | |
| 9 | Part of the sole of the back leg stepping on the ground | [ ] OK<br>[ ] OTHER<br>_____ | 200<br>0 | |
| 10 | Direction of the back leg | [ ] OK<br>[ ] INWARDS<br>[ ] OUTWARDS | 100<br>0 | |
| 11 | Direction of the knee of the back leg | [ ] OK<br>[ ] INWARDS<br>[ ] OUTWARDS | 250<br>0<br>0 | |
| 12 | Condition of the knee of the back leg | [ ] OK<br>[ ] BENT<br>[ ] LOCKED | 400<br>200<br>0 | |

| No | Description | Results of Observation | Possible Score | Your Score |
|---|---|---|---|---|
| 13 | Condition of the hip of the back leg | [ ] OK<br>[ ] SWAYED<br>[ ] LAZY | 200<br>100<br>0 | |
| 14 | Hip and waist of the back leg | [ ] OK<br>[ ] PRESSURE | 400<br>0 | |
| 15 | Direction of the body | [ ] OK<br>[ ] TO THE LEFT<br>[ ] TO THE RIGHT | 200<br>0<br>0 | |
| 16 | Body language: chest | [ ] OK<br>[ ] TENSE<br>[ ] HUNCHED | 300<br>0<br>100 | |
| 17 | Body language: shoulders, neck and head | [ ] OK<br>[ ] TENSE<br>[ ] BENT | 250<br>0<br>100 | |
| 18 | Body weight in the middle between the left and right legs | [ ] OK<br>[ ] SLIGHTLY<br>[ ] ON ONE LEG<br>[ ] EXTREMELY SWAYED | 500<br>250<br>100<br>0 | |
| 19 | Front leg when swung forward | [ ] OK<br>[ ] OTHER | 250<br>0 | |

| No | Description | Results of Observation | Possible Score | Your Score |
|---|---|---|---|---|
| 20 | Front leg straight forward without being rotated | [ ] OK<br>[ ] INWARDS<br>[ ] OUTWARDS | 200<br>0<br>0 | |
| 21 | Sole of the front foot when stepping | [ ] OK<br>[ ] OTHER<br>_____ | 100<br>0 | |
| 22 | Body weight as the front foot steps | [ ] OK<br>[ ] OTHER<br>_____ | 300<br>0 | |
| 23 | Back leg as the front leg swings | [ ] OK<br>[ ] NOT RELAXED | 200<br>0 | |
| | **Total points for the right leg** | | | |

## TABLE OF WALKING MEASUREMENTS – LEFT LEG

| No | Description | Results of Observation | Possible Score | Your Score |
|----|-------------|------------------------|----------------|------------|
| 1 | Distance between front foot and back foot | [ ] OK<br>[ ] INSUFFICIENT<br>[ ] SLIGHT<br>[ ] LARGE<br>[ ] EXCESSIVE | 2500<br>1000<br>1000<br>250<br>0 | |
| 2 | Distance between left foot and right foot | [ ] OK<br>[ ] SLIGHT<br>[ ] LARGE | 2500<br>1000<br>0 | |
| 3 | Alignment between left and right hips | [ ] OK<br>[ ] NOT ALIGNED | 5000<br>0 | |
| 4 | Part of the sole of the front foot stepping on the ground | [ ] OK<br>[ ] OTHER<br>_____ | 200<br>0 | |
| 5 | Direction of the front leg | [ ] OK<br>[ ] INWARDS<br>[ ] OUTWARDS | 100<br>0<br>0 | |
| 6 | Direction of the knee of the front leg | [ ] OK<br>[ ] INWARDS<br>[ ] OUTWARDS | 250<br>0<br>0 | |

| No | Description | Results of Observation | Possible Score | Your Score |
|----|-------------|------------------------|----------------|------------|
| 7 | Condition of the knee of the front leg | [ ] OK<br>[ ] BENT<br>[ ] LOCKED | 400<br>200<br>0 | |
| 8 | Condition of the hip of the front leg | [ ] OK<br>[ ] LAZY<br>[ ] SWAYED | 200<br>100<br>0 | |
| 9 | Part of the sole of the back leg stepping on the ground | [ ] OK<br>[ ] OTHER<br>_____ | 200<br>0 | |
| 10 | Direction of the back leg | [ ] OK<br>[ ] INWARDS<br>[ ] OUTWARDS | 100<br>0 | |
| 11 | Direction of the knee of the back leg | [ ] OK<br>[ ] INWARDS<br>[ ] OUTWARDS | 250<br>0<br>0 | |
| 12 | Condition of the knee of the back leg | [ ] OK<br>[ ] BENT<br>[ ] LOCKED | 400<br>200<br>0 | |

| No | Description | Results of Observation | Possible Score | Your Score |
|----|-------------|------------------------|----------------|------------|
| 13 | Condition of the hip of the back leg | [ ] OK<br>[ ] SWAYED<br>[ ] LAZY | 200<br>100<br>0 | |
| 14 | Hip and waist of the back leg | [ ] OK<br>[ ] PRESSURE | 400<br>0 | |
| 15 | Direction of the body | [ ] OK<br>[ ] TO THE LEFT<br>[ ] TO THE RIGHT | 200<br>0<br>0 | |
| 16 | Body language: chest | [ ] OK<br>[ ] TENSE<br>[ ] HUNCHED | 300<br>0<br>100 | |
| 17 | Body language: shoulders, neck and head | [ ] OK<br>[ ] TENSE<br>[ ] BENT | 250<br>0<br>100 | |
| 18 | Body weight in the middle between the left and right legs | [ ] OK<br>[ ] SLIGHTLY<br>[ ] ON ONE LEG<br>[ ] EXTREMELY SWAYED | 500<br>250<br>100<br>0 | |
| 19 | Front leg when swung forward | [ ] OK<br>[ ] OTHER<br>_____ | 250<br>0 | |

| No | Description | Results of Observation | Possible Score | Your Score |
|----|-------------|------------------------|----------------|------------|
| 20 | Front leg straight forward without being rotated | [ ] OK<br>[ ] INWARDS<br>[ ] OUTWARDS | 200<br>0<br>0 | |
| 21 | Sole of the front foot when stepping | [ ] OK<br>[ ] OTHER<br>_____ | 100<br>0 | |
| 22 | Body weight as the front foot steps | [ ] OK<br>[ ] OTHER<br>_____ | 300<br>0 | |
| 23 | Back leg as the front leg swings | [ ] OK<br>[ ] NOT RELAXED | 200<br>0 | |
| | **Total points for the left leg** | | | |

## CALCULATION OF POINTS AND RESULTS OF YOUR EVALUATION

| | |
|---|---|
| Total points for the right leg | |
| Total points for the left leg | |
| Total points for both legs **(Results of your evaluation)** | |

The allocation of points is based on the extent of the benefits or the negative effects of each matter being evaluated. After calculating the total points for both legs, review your evaluation results with reference to the **Table of Quality of Walk** below.

## TABLE OF QUALITY OF WALK

| Your Point Range | Description |
| --- | --- |
| 25,000 – 30,000 | **Excellent**<br>can improve body shape and overall health if you let the adjustments happen |
| 20,000 – 25,000 | **Good**<br>can improve body shape and overall health in a limited way if you let the adjustments happen |
| 15,000 – 20,000 | **OK** |
| 10,000 – 15,000 | **Not So Good**<br>can have negative effects on body shape and overall health |
| 5,000 – 10,000 | **Bad**<br>a lot of negative effects on body shape and overall health |
| 0 – 5,000 | **Very Bad**<br>very harmful to body and overall health |

# Chapter 6
## Mistakes Caused by Other Factors

As previously discussed, footwear with thick but soft soles will tend to cause the body weight to concentrate on one side of the sole of the foot, that is inwards, outwards, to the front or the back. Apart from such footwear, there are also other types of footwear that may potentially cause problems in the way of walking, the legs, or even the body as a whole.

However, it is important to remember that footwear is only one of the reasons someone might walk in an improper manner. There are also many other aspects which could cause problems in walking. In this regard, we will discuss these various issues in this chapter, so you may recognise and avoid them.

### FOOTWEAR
Generally, the types of footwear which may cause problems in the way we walk, our legs and our body are as follows:

### High-Heeled Shoes
Our body was not designed to function properly with high heels. In *Illustration 37*, you are able to observe how the bones

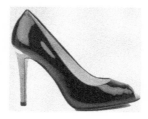

*Illustration 37: High-heeled shoes*

of the legs are extremely bent whilst wearing high heels. The body weight is also supported only by the pad of the foot and therefore is not spread throughout the whole sole of the foot as it should be. Prolonged wear can cause permanent damage and deformity in our feet and legs, alter our posture and natural spine alignment, damaging toe nails, worsen bunions and increase the risk of arthritis.

## Footwear with Thick and Soft Soles

Footwear with thick and soft soles may well feel comfortable, however you must ensure that the soles of the shoes are not too soft. If they are too soft, even when standing normally the body weight will tend to fall to one side and cause problems in the long run.

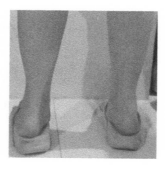

*Illustration 38: Effects of footwear with overly soft soles*

## Footwear with Uneven Soles

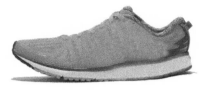

*Illustration 39: Footwear with uneven soles*

Many shoes, especially modern shoes, have soles that curve upwards. This will cause the sole of the foot to not be able to step properly and evenly as it should *(see Illustration 39)*.

## Footwear with Soles that are too Thin

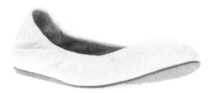

*Illustration 40: Footwear with soles that are too thin*

Some footwear are also constructed with extremely thin soles to make them lightweight. Although it is light, it is not ideal because the soles do serve an important function in absorbing the impact against the ground or floor when walking *(see Illustration 40)*.

## Flip-Flops/Thongs/Sandals

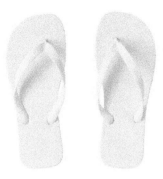

*Illustration 41: Flip-Flops/thongs/sandals*

According to American Podiatric Medical Association long term flip-flop wearers can suffer foot pain due to lack of arch support, tendinitis, and even sprained ankles. Flip-flops tend to overwork the leg muscles as the foot needs to be able to "hold" them. In addition, as we take our steps in such footwear, the soles of our feet are not able to work properly and naturally.

## Footwear with Worn Out Soles

If the soles of our footwear are worn out, either on the inside or outside part that directly touches the ground, the soles of our feet will not be able to step on the surface in an even manner as it should. When we walk with such footwear, the consequences are even worse.

Although the damage to the sole of the footwear tends to happen because of our improper way of walking, if we persist in wearing the same footwear, it will cause additional problems. Accordingly, if you happen to have such footwear, it is recommended you do not continue to wear them *(see Illustration 42)*.

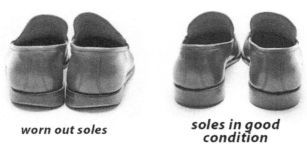

**worn out soles**          **soles in good condition**

*Illustration 42: Shoes with worn out soles*

## OTHER FACTORS

There are other factors which directly influence the way we walk, our legs and the health of our body, including:

1.  Placing a wallet in the back pocket.
2.  Carrying a bag on one shoulder.

### 1. Placing a Wallet in the Back Pocket

A habit of placing a wallet in the back pocket *(as shown in Illustration 43)* is a common habit for men. I myself had also done the same for many years, since the first time I owned a wallet in high school. However, I stopped doing this when I read an article, several years after graduating university. The article explained that by placing a wallet in our back pocket we will put pressure on the hip bone when we sit down. If this continues for an extended period of time, this pressure will also affect the spine and compress the sciatic nerve therefore affecting the health of our body negatively.

### 2. Carrying a Bag on One Shoulder

Carrying a bag on one shoulder as shown in the below illustration is common amongst women. Many women consider that carrying a bag on one shoulder is more comfortable and stylish. However, the results of many studies indicate that carrying a bag on one shoulder has a negative impact on health as the bag directly places pressure on the shoulder bone which is directly connected to the spine.

This burden on the shoulder bone will automatically have an effect on the spine which will therefore impact the whole body. It is preferable to hold the bag in your hand compared to carrying it on the shoulder. Although the bag may weigh the same, holding it will reduce the pressure on our shoulder.

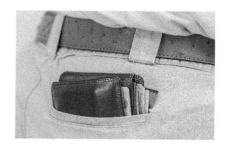

*Illustration 43: Placing a wallet in the back pocket*

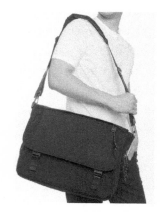

*Illustration 44: Carrying a bag on one shoulder*

# Chapter 7
## Secrets of Natural Walking® (SONW)

Secrets of Natural Walking® (SONW) is a natural method that invites us to recognise how we should walk naturally. As we have previously discussed, the human body is equipped with the ability to heal itself naturally. It is us who block this natural ability to the point that it ceases to function. Simultaneously, we also use our body in an improper manner which ultimately results in the body being unable to repair itself.

Regrettably, most humans do use their body in an improper manner in their daily lives. Because of this, correcting the way we walk will automatically restore many of the natural abilities inherent in our body. So, SONW may also be referred to as a natural therapy to straighten the spine, heal joint and bone problems and to reactivate the natural healing abilities of the body. Perhaps this may sound rather farfetched, however it is the reality.

*SONW may also be referred to as a natural therapy to straighten the spine, heal joint and bone problems and to reactivate the natural healing abilities of the body.*

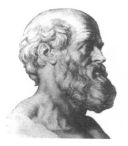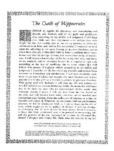

*Illustration 45: Hippocrates and the Hippocratic Oath*

Some of you may be wondering whether the idea of walking as a means of healing the body is a new idea? Not at all. Do you know about Hippocrates? Hippocrates lived in the Classical Greece era, around 460-377 BC *(see Illustration 45)*. He is famously known as the Father of Modern Medicine. Every physician in the world, when taking an oath would take the Hippocratic Oath. So, would you consider Hippocrates to be someone who understands the human body and health? As the Father of Modern Medicine, it should be so. Are you aware that Hippocrates stated that: "Walking is the best medicine" As the Father of Modern Medicine, certainly Hippocrates is someone who knows the secrets of healing the human body and the secret has been revealed clearly, that is "walking". Certainly, what is meant here is to walk properly which will allow us to reap many health benefits.

If we walk properly, then naturally:

- Joints, hips, spine, etc. will revert to their proper position.
- The meridians and reflexology zones will be stimulated and unblocked.
- Reactivation of the natural healing systems.
- Healing of internal diseases.
- Improvement of health, energy and stamina.
- The whole body will be more sculpted and toned *(see Illustration 46)*.

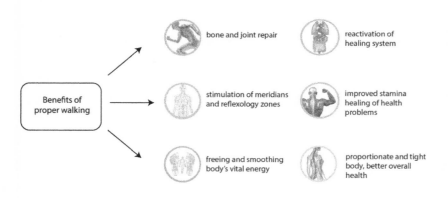

*Illustration 46: The whole body will be more sculpted and toned*

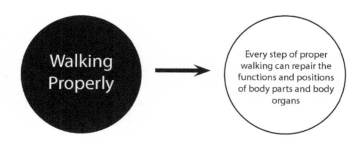

*Illustration 47: Benefits of walking properly*

So, if we walk properly, the bad habits we have carried all this time which reduce or halt the natural healing abilities of our body will be stopped. With SONW, we will end the causes of many problems and illnesses. These extraordinary abilities inherent in our body as a gift from our Creator will automatically function again and in this regard, every step taken using this method will correct the position and function of the bones, joints and internal organs of the body *(see **Illustration 47**)*.

# Chapter 8
## Basic Understanding of Secrets of Natural Walking®

You may be wondering: are we not already walking in a natural way? We do not use any equipment or tools to walk so automatically we are walking naturally, right?

If we see this from the perspective of the utilisation of walking aids (other than footwear), we would arrive at that conclusion. However, if we look deeper, what we have considered as natural is not actually natural at all. As I have touched on repeatedly, look at how the legs, hips and various body parts sway from left to right even though we are only walking forwards. Noting that these aspects are just the ones perceived by sight. There are many other issues that may not be perceptible by sight but nevertheless show that we do not walk naturally. Let us explore the causes of the mistakes that make us walk unnaturally.

## CAUSES OF THE MISTAKES

What will be discussed here is different compared to what was discussed previously in **Chapter 5**. In that chapter we discussed the various types of mistakes that are commonly found. Now, we will discuss the causes of those mistakes. Generally, the basic causes of these mistakes are as follows:

- Being in a hurry: controlling the whole body and even pulling the body or leg forwards.
- Habit of putting pressure on the body, including both legs, as a consequence of not being relaxed enough.
  - Laziness. This laziness may be exhibited only on a particular part of the body or a combination of several parts.
  - Lazy feet: the feet are directed all over the place or are being dragged.
  - Lazy knees: the knees are still bent or locked.
  - Lazy hips: the hips are still being swayed and the body weight is placed on one side of the body.
  - Lazy upper part of the body: folded stomach, back or shoulder hunched forward.
- External factors, for example what has been discussed in **Chapter 6**, such as wearing improper footwear, placing a wallet in the back pocket or carrying a bag on one shoulder.

## WALKING NATURALLY

After observing the causes of these mistakes, let us review the very basic matters to be able to understand the correct way of walking. In essence, to allow our body to function naturally. Remember again that we are discussing something out of the ordinary. Most techniques are of human creation and therefore learning these techniques is to learn how to control the body to move in accordance with the particular technique. However, here we are discussing something vastly different, that is to allow our body to function naturally. So, the most important key is to let go of the control over our whole body, including:

- Letting go of the control over our body, while being relaxed but not lazy. The method is as follows:
  - Hip joints to rotate naturally.
  - Left and right hips must always be naturally parallel, from the left and right side, front and back and above and below.
  - Body weight in the middle (between left foot and right foot).
- Both legs and whole body directed straight forward, because we walk in a forward direction. There is no part of our body moving sideways or bending.
- Sole of the foot to step on the earth naturally, just in accordance with the gravitational pull of the earth, without being pushed or forced, but also not being overly controlled.

*Natural means to let go of the control over our body so that the whole body may function naturally, whilst being relaxed but not lazy.*

## Experiment 8:
## Swinging one leg forward

To help you understand better, let us try a simple experiment. We will step forward with one leg. To simplify the discussion, please step forward with your right leg. Repeat it several times while feeling:

Are you actually swinging your right leg? Many people do not actually swing their leg but drag or push their leg forward *(see Illustration 48)*. There are others who add an additional movement, such as pushing after swinging their leg, even though the best is to just simply swing their leg forward.

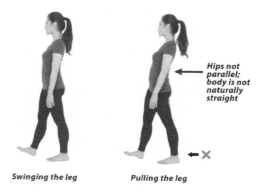

Swinging the leg          Pulling the leg

*Illustration 48: Swinging the leg*

Are you swinging the whole right leg forward? Some people only swing the sole of their foot. Over the long term, these people tend to find their thighs becoming lazier and looser. People who swing only the sole of their foot in an overpowering manner will also experience excessive pressure on their knees. There are also people who only swing their thighs, causing their thighs and knees to be lifted higher than it should be. Upon lowering, their feet will stomp on the ground with more force than it should. This will cause negative consequences on the knees, feet and whole body.

Are you swinging your right leg directly straight forward? There are also many people who swing their leg inwards or outwards first before changing direction to face forward. **See Illustration 49** and **Illustration 50** for clarification. You may suggest that this does not matter as the end result is the same, because the right leg ends up being swung forward anyway. However, although it is true that the right leg ends up at the desired location, if you swing the right leg inwards or outwards first before directing it forward, the muscles and muscle fibres in your leg have rotated in a different direction. This causes the leg to no longer be straight in the way it should be.

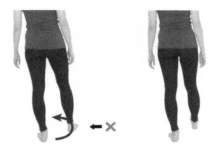

*Illustration 49: Swinging the leg outwards before forwards*

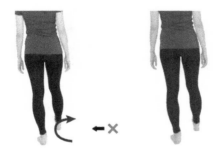

*Illustration 50: Swinging the leg inwards before forwards*

Is the sole of your foot directed sufficiently normally forward or directed too much outwards or inwards? The direction of the sole of your foot is also an important factor. Because of this, it is essential to know whether the sole of your foot is directed sufficiently normally forward.

Exactly after swinging your leg, how relaxed is your back leg *(see Illustration 51)* Are you tensing your left leg? Many people usually tense their back leg when swinging their front leg.

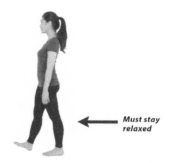

Illustration 51: Back leg must stay relaxed

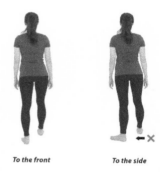

To the front          To the side

Illustration 52: Back leg must continue to be directed forwards

Is the sole of your back foot still facing the same direction? For some people, when they step forward, their back foot tends to be pulled in such a way that the direction of the sole of the back foot changes. Usually the foot will open outwards as seen in **Illustration 52.**

If you are sufficiently relaxed, after swinging your right leg, your left and right hips should be quite parallel. However, for most people their hips are not parallel. So, when swinging their right leg, the right hip will tend to be pulled forward *(see Illustration 53).* This is not ideal for our hips and spine and will also have broad implications for the health of the whole body.

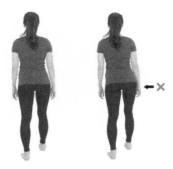

**Parallel Hips**          **Hips pulled forwards**

*Illustration 53: Hips parallel after leg swing (proper) VS. hip pulled forward (improper)*

Is your stride too wide? If your stride is too wide, your right hip will be too far forward relative to your left hip *(see Illustration 54).* Your right hip will be pulled forward too much and cause excessive pressure on your lower spine.

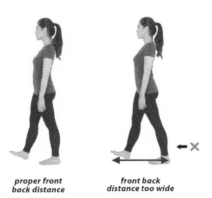

**proper front**          **front back**
**back distance**          **distance too wide**

*Illustration 54: Proper front-back distance VS. a stride that is too wide*

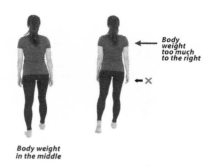

*Illustration 55: Body weight centered (proper) VS. body weight to one side (improper)*

Is your body weight sufficiently in between the left and right sections of your body? If your body weight is being supported too much by the right side of the body, it is highly likely that you are throwing your legs when you walk *(see Illustration 55).*

Does your body lean too far forward? Those people who are too much in a rush or are often in a rush will usually overly control their body when walking. Consequently, their whole body feels as if it is brought forward as fast as possible *(see Illustration 56).*

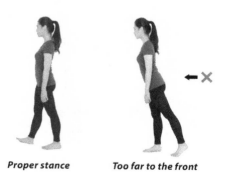

*Illustration 56: Proper stance VS. improper stance*

Based on this discussion we are able to observe our numerous bad habits in just one step. We may be walking improperly merely to achieve a certain style, but evidently it causes problems with the shape and/or health of our body. Moreover, the points discussed do not even cover all the mistakes that might exist in just one step.

# Chapter 9
## Walking Method Improvement and the Stages of Changes to the Body

After reading the previous chapters, you may be somewhat confused. Perhaps you might have formed a view that there is much to learn to be able to walk properly. Subsequently, you may consider that improving the way you walk may be rather difficult.

### CHANGING THE WAY YOU WALK IS NOT DIFFICULT

Walking is something we all have been doing since a young age. We do it in our daily lives to the point that it is a habit. Notwithstanding this, mistakes in the way that we walk may be corrected relatively easily as we are not talking about how to walk in the perfect way. The aim is to reduce or stop our bad habits. Quite a number of people have experienced the immediate benefits from the first day that they started to correct the way they walk. Because of this, do not worry, the most important thing is that you are serious in wanting to change the way that you walk. The easiest way to change the way you walk is through the following steps:

1. Learning the proper way of walking.
2. Practicing the proper way of walking routinely.
3. Trying to correct the way you walk in your daily life.

> *Mistakes in the way that we walk may be corrected relatively easily as we are not talking about how to walk in the perfect way. The aim is to reduce or stop our bad habits.*

If you carry out the above, especially point 3, in time you will realise how the way you walk has changed. The most interesting aspect of starting to walk properly is that your overall health will have changed too. As long as you are doing it every day without forcing yourself you will realise that your health has improved significantly.

If you are still confused, perhaps we can use an example. Take someone who is learning a foreign language by attending a course to learn that foreign language. This person however never practices the foreign language outside course hours. After one year, how fluent would this person be in the foreign language? If you have experienced it yourself or know of someone like this, you will certainly know that this person would not be very fluent in the foreign language. One year is a sufficient length of time but even with regular classes, without practice the results will be limited.

On the other hand, if another person attends the same foreign language course, committing the same amount of formal study time each week, but always practices the language even outside course hours, in just a few months this person will most likely be quite fluent. Although both these people may learn from the same instructor, have the same study materials and spend the exact same amount of time in class, their ability will be vastly different because the second person is diligent in practicing. Practice is a vital part in learning any skill.

With this example, after you have learnt the keys in correcting the way you walk, you will only need to do the following important thing, that is to practice and practice. In time, you will improve significantly and reap the benefits. The shape of your body, your health and other matters will improve naturally too.

However, although in this book I spell out the instructions and various descriptions that are quite complete, if you wish to obtain the best results then you must treat SONW as a skill/method/technique. Additionally, to obtain the best results it will be helpful to obtain direct guidance from someone with experience in SONW. You will be able to join workshops taught by trained and certified instructors. This information is provided in **Chapter 20**.

## STAGES OF CHANGES TO THE BODY

In changing the way you walk, your body will start to also change automatically. Usually the first changes will initially be felt in relation to problems with the joints, hips and spine. If you have such problems, in a few days to a few weeks you will be able to feel clear changes.

Subsequently, changes will happen on the muscles and the shape of the body. You will start to feel your leg, chest and other muscles tighten. The shape of your body starts to change. However, during this phase usually it is the females who might be concerned. Females who prefer a slim figure will feel anxious when there are parts of the body that start to "enlarge", such as their breasts becoming more voluptuous and their backsides becoming "fuller". But with continued practice, all these changes are actually very good because usually females who experience these changes are females with "flat" bodies. Conversely for females who have a "loose" or "excessive" body, they will generally feel immediate changes that are more according to their hopes in that various parts of their body becoming tighter and more sculpted.

Indeed, the most interesting part of SONW is that everything happens in accordance to its proper proportions. Those people with loose bodies become tighter and more toned. Those people with a "flat" body become fuller. Let's just see, aren't the bodies of females and males naturally different? Although we will not be able to fully understand our bodies, it is all the greatest gift from our Creator. By letting our body work naturally, including the process of healing and change, all the best things will happen so beautifully.

So, if you practice routinely, in just a few months many changes will occur. Various ailments will be cured, there will be improvements in the body shape, increased stamina, calmer mind and so on. Regrettably, for many people once their ailments or problems disappear, they are no longer motivated to continue practicing. If the way they walk is proper the reparations to the whole body will continue to function. However, if the old bad habits are still there then the condition of the body will decline again.

On the other hand, if you continue to practice diligently, the changes that have happened on your body will not stop at just these interesting things that we have discussed. More changes to your body will continue to occur, even beyond the expectations of many people. These changes are beyond what is attainable by those people who practice at the gym routinely in relation to the body and muscle shape. Simultaneously, the changes will also happen to the internal organs. These organs become healthier, fresher and function better. Many people who suffer from high cholesterol levels, high blood glucose levels and decreased kidney function have recovered. They are fresher, more energetic and even have more vitality compared to their younger selves. The body's endurance and stamina will also improve significantly. There are people who would usually already be shivering being in a room with a temperature of 24 degrees Celsius. However, after diligently practicing SONW for a few months, they are relaxed in normal clothing when being in a room with a temperature of 22 degrees Celsius *(see Illustration 57).*

So, if someone is diligent in practicing SONW, over a long period of time the ageing process will stop or even reverse. You might not believe what I have just stated however the majority of the ageing process happens not because the body is consumed by age, but because of the improper use and abuse of the body *(see Illustration 58).*

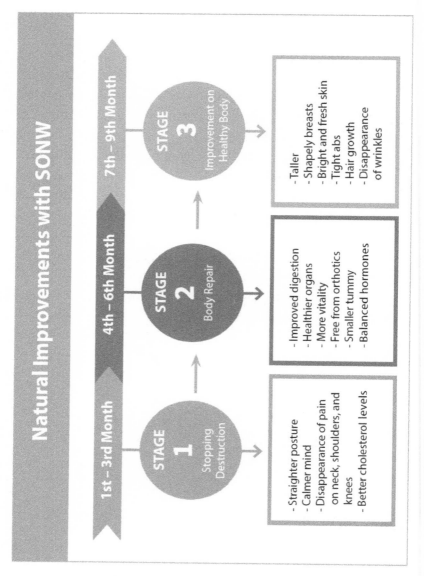

*Illustration 57: Natural healing with SONW*

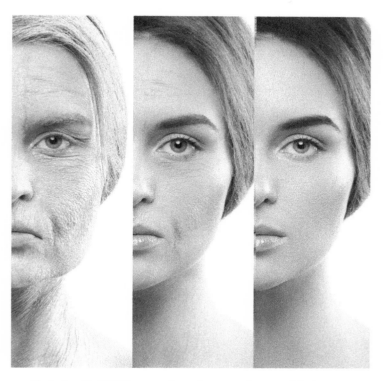

*Illustration 58: SONW reverses the ageing process because of the improper use of the body*

# Chapter 10
## Basic Understanding of Natural Walking

To be able to walk naturally, apart from being aware of the basic principles as discussed in **Chapter 8**, you must also understand the following important basics:

- Distance between left foot and right foot
- Distance between front foot and back foot
- How to place the sole of the foot on the ground
- Walking straight
- The whole body directed straight forward, not allowing it to sway or bend

However, as previously discussed, although all of the above are extremely important, it all has to happen naturally. We must let go of our control over the whole body. It all has to happen in a relaxed, but not lazy manner.

Prior to going into further detail, it is best to first discuss the terminology to be utilised in describing the various parts of our leg to avoid any misunderstanding. In *Illustration 59*, you are able to see the parts of the leg we will be referring to in the following discussion:

- Knee
- Heel
- Pad of the foot
- Ball of the foot

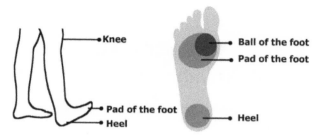

*Illustration 59: General parts of the legs and feet*

Now that we are clear in relation to the different parts of the leg and feet, let us discuss the vital basics in SONW.

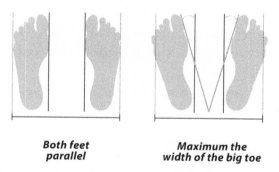

**Both feet parallel**

**Maximum the width of the big toe**

*Illustration 60: Distance and alignment of the left foot and right foot*

## DISTANCE BETWEEN LEFT FOOT AND RIGHT FOOT

As previously discussed in **Chapter 5,** *Illustration 31* shows that the ideal distance between the left foot and right foot is to be the same as the width of the person's hip bones. This is natural and makes logical sense. If our legs are sufficiently in line with our hip bone, the soles of our feet will be even against the ground. By contrast, if the distance between the left foot and right foot is narrower or wider than the width of our hip bones, there will be a tendency for us to step inwards or outwards. If this happens, our knees will also bend inwards or outwards, affecting the shape of our legs. However, these effects described are only superficial as the whole body and our overall health will also be negatively impacted.

Closely related to the issue of the distance between the left foot and right foot, you must also be aware of the alignment of your feet. Both soles of the feet should be relatively straight and parallel, although it does not necessarily need to be perfectly parallel. The feet are allowed to "open" with a maximum width of the big toe *(see Illustration 60)*. If the position of the feet opens more than the width of the big toe, you will need to slowly pull the front part of your sole to correct it.

## DISTANCE BETWEEN THE FRONT FOOT AND BACK FOOT

In **Chapter 5** and *Illustration 30*, the optimal distance between the front foot and back foot while you are walking normally is ½ the length of the sole of your foot, marked as X, equal to ½ L.

## HOW TO PLACE THE SOLE OF THE FOOT ON THE GROUND

In placing the sole of the foot, we must place the heel on the ground first. Then the front part may be placed, that is the pad of the foot *(see Illustration 61)*. If you are relaxed (as you should be), automatically it will not just be the pad of your foot that touches the ground, but also all of your toes. As previously noted, when stepping, the entire outer, inner, front and back parts of the foot must be even as shown in **Illustration 62**.

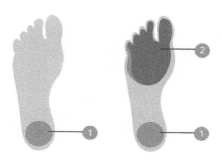

*Illustration 61: How to place the sole of the foot on the ground*

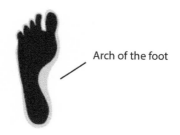

Arch of the foot

*Illustration 62: Sole of the foot stepping evenly on the ground*

In stepping, it should also be remembered that everything must happen naturally. So, do it while being relaxed, slowly, without pressing. Please note that slowly does not mean so slow as if you are placing an egg on a hard surface. If the movement is too slow, it will cause you to hold and control your feet and consequently you will not be able to relax.

## WALKING HAS TO BE STRAIGHT

As it can be seen in ***Illustration 63***, it is clear how some people do not walk in a straight line. We should naturally be walking in a relatively straight manner.

## THE WHOLE BODY DIRECTED STRAIGHT FORWARD

Because we usually walk in a forward direction, our body should also move forwards. All movements that bring parts of our body sideways, to bend and so on are not natural and will have a negative impact on the related parts of the body and overall health.

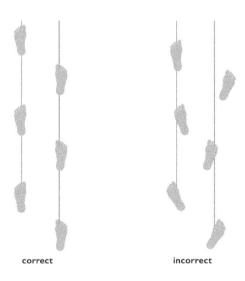

correct                    incorrect

*Illustration 63: Walking straight (proper) vs. not walking straight (improper)*

# Chapter 11
## 6 Basic Keys of Secrets of Natural Walking® (SONW)

In SONW, to help someone correct the way they walk, one step has been divided into six smaller parts. For simplicity, I will refer to these parts as "keys". Each SONW step is divided into six keys *(Illustration 64)*.

- **Key 1:** Swinging the Leg
- **Key 2:** Pumping the Pad of the Foot
- **Key 3:** Gliding while Rolling the Back Foot
- **Key 4:** Letting Adjustments Happen
- **Key 5:** Letting Go of Body Weight into the Earth
- **Key 6:** The Next Step

Although we refer to the existence of six keys, there are actually only three movements in SONW, which are:

- **Key 1:** Swinging the Leg
- **Key 2:** Pumping the Pad of the Foot
- **Key 3:** Body Gliding Forwards While Rolling the Back Foot

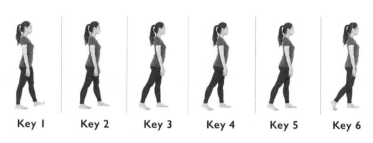

Key 1     Key 2     Key 3     Key 4     Key 5     Key 6

*Illustration 64: Keys 1-6 SONW*

**Key 4** is done while stationary, there is no movement at all. Same with **Key 5**. Whilst **Key 6** is essentially the same as **Key 1**.

Are the two keys with no movement part of walking more naturally? Why would we not move when we are walking? Perhaps you may find this puzzling. Let us consider briefly the function of these two keys, **Key 4** and **Key 5**.

**Key 4** is required because we intend to allow each step to change and repair the various parts of our body. So that this may occur, we must give it enough time. **Key 4** provides the time required for this repair and change to happen.

> *Although there are six keys, in terms of actual movements, there are actually only 3 movements:*
> *Key 1: Swinging the leg*
> *Key 2: Pumping the pad of the foot*
> *and Key 3: Gliding the body while rolling the back foot.*

If we have stopped or in other words are not moving in **Key 4**, why would we have **Key 5** which has no movement either? Although **Key 5** shares this similarity with **Key 4**, the function of **Key 5** is completely different to **Key 4**. **Key 5** aims to let go of the body weight into the earth. Why would we want to let go of our body weight into the earth? Without letting go of the body weight into the earth, our body weight will be unable to be connected to the earth properly. As I have mentioned several times previously, the evenness of the outer and inner parts and the front and back parts of the sole of the foot is vitally important. Without letting go of our body weight into the earth, we will tend to not step evenly on the surface of the earth. Because of this we need **Key 5**.

Although there is a differentiation between **Key 6** and **Key 1**, they are essentially the same and the proceeding movement is **Key 2** *(see **Illustration 65**)*. This is why the SONW method is said to actually only have three movements notwithstanding that the full movement consists of a total of six keys.

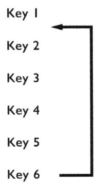

*Illustration 65: The use of keys in SONW*

If **Key 6** is so similar to **Key 1**, why was such a distinction made? This is because the starting position prior to taking the first step is extremely important (i.e. the distance between the left foot and right foot). Moving the leg properly when carrying out this first movement is also extremely important to train the muscles of the legs that were previously usually not engaged. Conversely, the muscles that we are not meant to use in daily life but were previously forced to be engaged may be relaxed. Because of this a distinction is made in relation to the first movement and especially labelled as **Key 1**.

For clarity, I will elaborate further in relation to each of the SONW keys to you. I will also provide further explanations, information on body weight and common mistakes made by people in each key.

# Chapter 12
## Key 1: Swinging the Leg

B ecause every key is a part of one step, broken down like this it is a simple movement. However, the real challenge is to change our habits, including rushing, holding the body or even being lazy and to correct them. We must allow the parts of our body to function naturally without a trace of laziness.

## INSTRUCTIONS

- Without shifting the body weight, swing your right leg forward so that the heel rests on the floor with the correct distance, your knee relaxed with the weight of your leg on your heel.
- Start with a different leg every day to ensure that both of your legs develop equally *(see Illustration 66)*.

## EXPLANATION

**Key 1** is a simple movement to swing the leg forward. The most significant difference compared to the usual habit in day-to-day walking is that the body weight is not immediately shifted to the front leg. In fact, the body weight remains on the back leg (with only a slight shift because of the movement of the front leg). The front foot carries only the weight of the front leg.

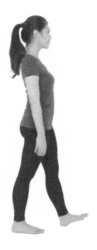

*Illustration 66: Key 1: Swinging the Leg*

## BODY WEIGHT

When the right leg is swung forward, *Illustration 67* shows the shift of the body weight prior to and following **Key 1**.

It is also important to remember that the body weight between the left and right legs must be maintained in the middle (in a sufficiently natural way). Note that it is natural for the body weight to initially shift slightly to the left prior to swinging the right leg forward. Subsequently, after **Key 1** is completed, the body weight reverts to the middle of the body between the left and right legs *(see Illustration 68)*.

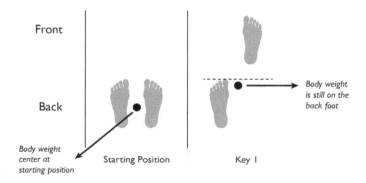

Illustration 67: Shifting of the body weight between the front foot and back
foot prior to and following Key 1: Swinging the Leg

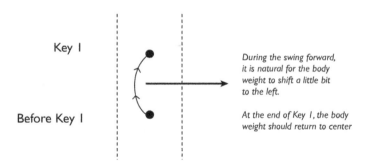

Illustration 68: Shifting of the body weight between the left foot and right foot
prior to and following Key 1: Swinging the Leg

## COMMON MISTAKES

1. Left and right hip not parallel
2. The knee is not relaxed and has a tendency to lock in the next steps.
3. Sole of the foot too close to the ground
4. Distance between the front foot and the back foot too close

5. Distance between the front foot and back foot too far
6. Slamming the heel
7. The body weight is placed too much on the front leg
8. Pulling down the front leg
9. Lifting the knees too high

To help you better understand, an explanation is given in relation to each one of these mistakes below.

## 1. LEFT AND RIGHT HIP NOT PARALLEL

If following **Key 1** your left and right hips are not parallel *(Illustration 69)*, it means you are not swinging your front leg properly, or otherwise your back leg is too stiff. At the very least there was a moment where you forcibly pushed your front leg forward.

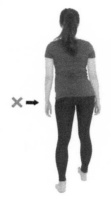

I have couched it in these terms because the condition of the legs and the way each person walks will not be exactly the same. Some people do not swing their front leg when stepping and instead they push. Some other people initially swing their front leg but then give an additional push too. This mistake may even be combined with a back

*Illustration 69:*
*Left and right*
*hips not parallel*

leg that is too stiff resulting in the hip joints and back leg not moving at all (and automatically being left behind in the movement).

## 2. THE KNEE IS NOT RELAXED AND HAS A TENDENCY TO LOCK IN THE NEXT STEPS.

If after **Key 1** the knee of your front leg is not relaxed *(Illustration 70)*, there is a significant tendency to lock your knees after the next key, **Key 2**. Because of this you must ensure your knees are sufficiently relaxed but also straight. If it is not straight, you will not obtain the optimal benefits of this SONW method.

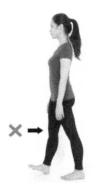

*Illustration 70: Knees not relaxed resulting in them being locked*

## 3. SOLE OF THE FOOT TOO CLOSE TO THE GROUND

If after **Key 1** the sole of your foot is too close to the ground *(Illustration 71)*, the weight of the leg would have already been divided between the heel and ball of the foot and there will be insufficient space to pump the pad of the foot properly. Because everything has to happen naturally, this insufficient amount of space will cause the body weight to be too far back when you perform **Key 2**. Ideally the body weight should be supported between the front and back legs.

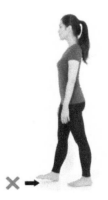

*Illustration 71: Sole of the foot too close to the ground*

## 4. DISTANCE BETWEEN THE FRONT FOOT AND BACK FOOT TOO CLOSE

The issue of the distance between the front foot and the back foot being too close (see *Illustration 72*) cannot actually be said to be a mistake.

By doing this there are no negative effects on the legs or body. However, with the distance between the front and back leg being too close the steps you take will not be able to give sufficient benefits to change and repair your body naturally.

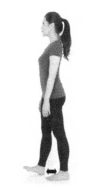

*Illustration 72: Distance between the front foot and the back foot too close*

## 5. DISTANCE BETWEEN FRONT FOOT AND THE BACK FOOT TOO FAR

Too far of a distance between the front foot and back foot *(Illustration 73)* may have a negative impact on your legs and body. If the distance is too wide but not excessive, the muscles in your legs will tend to be tenser in order to maintain the body's balance. Also, if the distance is too far, the hip of the front leg will tend to be pulled forward causing the left and right hips to no longer be parallel. As we have previously discussed, this is one of the mistakes which could potentially cause spinal problems.

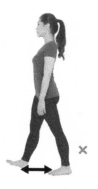

*Illustration 73: Distance between front foot and back foot too far.*

## 6. SLAMMING THE HEEL

The whole body, including the legs, should be utilised in a natural manner. Using the body naturally includes moving the body in a relaxed and smooth way, without pressing or slamming. If the heel is slammed on the ground *(see Illustration 74)*, the muscles of the front leg, especially the back part, will be tense. Even if you relax them subsequently, these muscles will usually not be able to relax naturally. This condition disturbs the adjustments and/or the other changes that are supposed to happen naturally in each step. A habit of slamming the heel can also have a negative impact on the heel bone and whole leg over the long term. Problems may then appear in relation to the heel bone or the related parts.

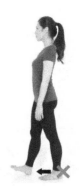

*Illustration 74:*
*Stomping the heel*

## 7. THE BODY WEIGHT IS PLACED TOO MUCH ON THE FRONT LEG

Similar to the previous mistake, slamming the heel, if the body weight is supported too much by the front leg *(see Illustration 75)*, the muscles of the front leg will over tighten. This mistake will disturb the adjustments or changes that are supposed to occur naturally in every step we take. The body weight should still be supported by the back leg, even though it will not be exactly in the middle of the back leg as shown in **Illustration 67**.

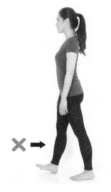

*Illustration 75: The Body weight is placed too much on the front leg*

## 8. PULLING DOWN THE FRONT LEG

For some people, this mistake is made during the process of swinging the leg. There are people who do not place their heel on the ground naturally when swinging the leg, but instead pull it downwards *(Illustration 76)*. This mistake will cause the same problem as slamming the heel because this movement will result in excessive pressure on the heel compared to if the heel is placed naturally on the ground. Although the majority of people who make this mistake do it because they lift their knee too high when swinging the leg, those people who do not lift their knee too high are not immune from this mistake either.

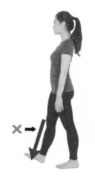

*Illustration 76: Pulling the front leg down*

## 9. LIFTING THE KNEES TOO HIGH

If you swing your leg naturally, that is in a relaxed manner, the whole leg together will swing forwards. However, if you lift your knee too high *(see Illustration 77)*, this is not swinging your leg naturally. By lifting the knee too high, when it comes time to be lowered you will most certainly make the mistake previously alluded to, that is pulling the front leg downwards. Based on the descriptions about the common mistakes made by people in **Key 1**, you will understand that it will affect **Key 2**. Poor execution of **Key 2** will also affect the

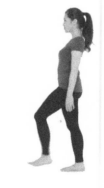

*Illustration 77: Lifting the knees too high*

subsequent keys. Because of this you must be able to master **Key 1** well before proceeding to **Key 2**.

Although I have given these nine examples of common mistakes this is not a comprehensive or complete list of mistakes that might be made in relation to **Key 1**. There are many other possibilities. However, complicated issues are usually not easily identified other than by those who are experienced in SONW.

# Chapter 13
## Key 2: Pumping the Pad of the Foot

As its name suggests, **Key 2** is a simple movement, consisting of just pumping the pad of the front foot. Because this movement is done while being relaxed, the whole body just follows forward. With this, the body weight is now supported between the front foot and back foot *(see Illustration 79)* and also between the left foot and right foot.

### INSTRUCTIONS

- With the whole leg directed straight forward, pump the pad of your foot. The knee will be straight but not locked.
- At this point, your body is quite straight and relaxed with the weight of the body somewhere around the front and back foot.
- Ensure the part of the foot that is pumping is the pad of the foot and the body is not too far forward. *(see Illustration 78)*.

## EXPLANATION

Remember, the instruction given is to pump the pad of the foot while being relaxed. So, this does not mean you should press the sole of the foot or press the whole leg either. In practice, this movement may also be said to be lowering the sole of the foot to the ground in a relaxed manner. However, if I were to give the following instruction, that is to "lower the sole of the foot to the ground in a relaxed manner", some people would tend to only lower the sole of their foot without letting their whole body adjust as well, including the shifting of the body weight from the back foot to between the back foot and the front foot. Because of this the instruction is to "pump the pad of the foot".

Because you are relaxed, the whole body should also follow so that the body weight starts to shift from the back foot to the middle of the body. However, because this occurs as an effect of pumping the pad of the foot and as the pad is actually special, there will not be any jarring motion transmitted to our body or even our legs.

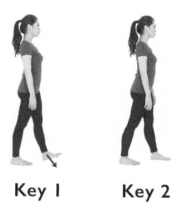

## Key 1          Key 2

*Illustration 78: Key 2: Pumping the Pad of the Foot*

## BODY WEIGHT

Pay attention to *Illustration 79* and *Illustration 80*. After **Key 2**, it can be seen how the body weight that was previously supported more by the back foot (between the front foot and back foot), now has shifted completely to the middle. Simultaneously, the body weight between the left foot and right foot after completing **Key 1** is also still in the middle. So, the body weight is supported in between the left foot and right foot and in between the front foot and back foot. I would usually refer to this condition as the body weight being in the "center".

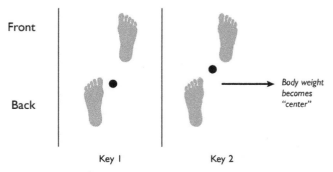

*Illustration 79: Shifting of the body weight between the front foot and back foot before and after Key 2: Pumping the Pad of the Foot*

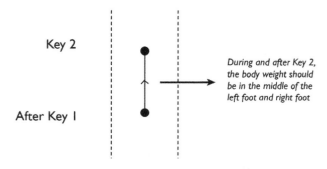

*Illustration 80: Shifting of the body weight between the left foot and right foot before and after Key 2: Pumping the Pad of the Foot*

## COMMON MISTAKES:

1.  Bringing the body forward at the same time as the foot
2.  The body is too far forward
3.  Slamming the pad of the foot
4.  Pumping with the whole leg
5.  The left and right hips are not parallel
6.  The hip is directed diagonally
7.  Only the pad of the foot is pressed to the floor
8.  The knee is not straight forward
9.  The thigh is not straight forward
10. The front foot opens too wide
11. The back foot opens too wide

For your better understanding, please find an explanation for each of these mistakes below.

## 1. BRINGING THE BODY FORWARD AT THE SAME TIME AS THE FOOT

It is indeed our habit to walk in a rush in order to reach the desired destination. Because of this, every time we move our leg, our body tends to also move forward together *(Illustration 81)*. Contrast this to the fact that at this stage we should only just be stepping with the sole of our foot in a natural way. Of course, the body weight will shift slightly forward but only to the point between the front foot and back foot. The body weight should not have shifted to the front foot at this stage.

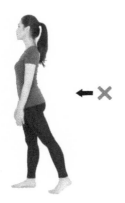

*Illustration 81:*
*Bringing the body*
*forward at the same*
*time as the foot.*

## 2. THE BODY IS TOO FAR FORWARD

For some people in doing this key, although their body weight is sufficiently in between the front foot and back foot, their body is too far forward *(Illustration 82)*. In this condition, the body weight will not truly be in between the front foot and back foot. There will therefore be excessive pressure on the hips. This pressure will increase in the next key when such a mistake has been made.

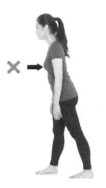

*Illustration 82: The body is too far forward*

## 3. SLAMMING THE PAD OF THE FOOT

When pumping the pad of the foot, the pad of the foot should be lowered onto the ground naturally, relaxed and certainly not in a slamming motion *(Illustration 83)*. If the pad of the foot is moved in a slamming motion or is being dragged, the muscles of the front leg will be tense and place pressure on the hips.

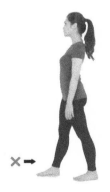

*Illustration 83: Slamming the pad of the foot*

## 4. PUMPING WITH THE WHOLE LEG

This key should only be a simple movement of the sole of the foot to pump the pad of the foot. However, some people instead pump their whole leg to push the sole of the foot downwards *(Illustration 84)*. Although it may appear to be similar, the muscles utilised are completely different. Similar to the previous mistake, that is to thump the pad of the foot, this mistake will cause the muscles of the front leg to be tense and place pressure on the hips.

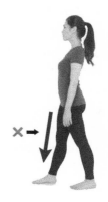

*Illustration 84: Pumping with the whole leg*

## 5. THE LEFT AND RIGHT HIPS ARE NOT PARALLEL

The mistake of moving the whole leg may cause an even worse mistake. If at the moment the whole front leg is moved or pushed to the ground and the back leg is insufficiently relaxed, the hip of the front leg will be pulled forward causing it to no longer be parallel with the other hip *(Illustration 85)*. As discussed several times previously, hips that are not parallel may cause significant problems with the spine, body posture and overall health.

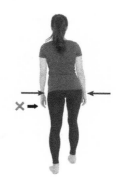

*Illustration 85: Left and right hips are not parallel*

## 6. THE HIP IS DIRECTED DIAGONALLY

Similar to the previous mistake, that is the "left and right hips not being parallel", some people have the tendency to sway their hips when moving the front leg (Illustration 86). Consequently, other than the hips not being parallel, the front hip is also "twisted".

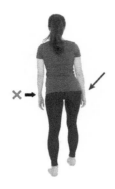

*Illustration 86: Swaying the hips when pumping the pad of the foot*

## 7. ONLY THE PAD OF THE FOOT IS PRESSED TO THE FLOOR

Previously I have noted that some people will pump their whole leg to press the pad of their foot to the ground. Conversely, there are others who just pump the pad of their foot but at the same time hold the rest of their body. Consequently, the rest of the body does not move in unison with the placement of the pad of the foot on the ground *(Illustration 87)*. This kind of movement will produce excessive pressure on the muscles within the front foot and even to the hips.

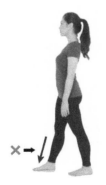

*Illustration 87: Only the pad of the foot pressing on the ground*

## 8. THE KNEE IS NOT STRAIGHT FORWARD

This mistake is somewhat similar to the previous mistake, that is "pumping the whole leg". This happens because the person does not limit the movement to a simple pumping of the pad of the foot but also moves the knees. Further to make matters worse, the knee which is supposed to be straight is pushed outwards or inwards *(Illustration 88* or also see *Illustration 35).*

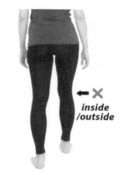

*Illustration 88: Knees not directed straight forward*

## 9. THE THIGH IS NOT STRAIGHT FORWARD

Similar to the mistake of "the knee is not straight forward", there are also people who when pumping the pad of their foot will also move their thighs. The thighs being moved may shift outwards or inwards *(Illustration 89).*

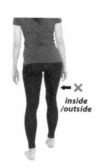

*Illustration 89: Thighs not directed straight forward*

## 10. THE FRONT FOOT OPENS TOO WIDE

In performing the pumping motion of the sole of the front foot that should be quite simple, some people will turn their foot outwards prior to pumping the pad of the front foot to the ground *(Illustration 90)*.

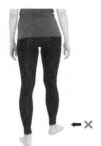

*Illustration 90: Front foot turning outward/opens too wide*

## 11. THE BACK FOOT OPENS TOO WIDE

There are also people who allow their body to move naturally when pumping the pad of their foot but doing so in an excessive manner. Consequently, the back foot also turns to an open position when the proper position is for the foot to be directed straight forward *(Illustration 91)*.

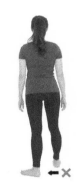

*Illustration 91: Back foot turns outward/opens too wide*

# Chapter 14
## Key 3: Gliding the Body While Rolling the Back Foot

Our body weight will shift completely to the front foot in Key 3 *(Illustration 92, Illustration 93* and *Illustration 94)*. Because both soles of the feet do not move from their respective positions, this movement does not cause any jarring motions.

### INSTRUCTIONS

Let your body glide forwards just until it is aligned with the front leg, in the process let:
- the left and right sections stay straight and parallel
- let your spine be aligned naturally
- let the back foot roll gradually
- until the body is in line with the front leg.

At this point, your front knee will be quite straight but not locked. The pad and the ball of your back foot will support your body weight but do not push forwards.

## EXPLANATION

As I have previously explained, you must have performed **Key 1** and **Key 2** properly to be able to do **Key 3** properly.

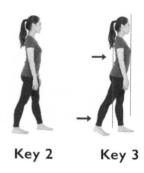

**Key 2**          **Key 3**

*Illustration 92: Key 3: Gliding the Body While Rolling the Back Foot*

**Key 3** is done together between the front and back leg. Do not worry about how many percent you must allocate to each leg because we are not learning about a man-made technique but rather a natural movement.

The vital issue here is to ensure the left and right hips are kept parallel during and after this key is completed.

This is a rather interesting key because usually people who are new to SONW tend to initially experience difficulties with this key. However, after practicing for some time, **Key 3** can be performed with relative ease.

## BODY WEIGHT

The body weight which was previously positioned in the center, that is in between the left foot and right foot and also in between the front foot and back foot, now shifts to the front foot. However, the body weight will still be located between the left foot and right foot *(Illustration 93 and 94)*.

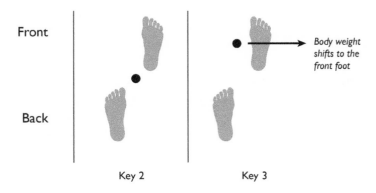

*Illustration 93: Shifting of the body weight between the front foot and back foot before and after Key 3: Gliding the Body While Rolling the Back Foot*

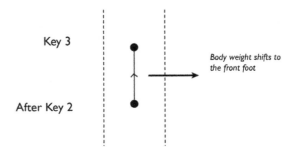

*Illustration 94: Shifting of the body weight between the left foot and right foot before and after Key 3: Gliding the Body While Rolling the Back Foot*

## COMMON MISTAKES:

1. The back foot is not rolled, but pushed.
2. The body is too far forward beyond the front foot.
3. The back foot is not supporting the body.
4. Looking downwards.
5. Body weight is not evenly distributed on the front foot.

To help you better understand, an explanation is given in relation to each one of these mistakes below.

## 1. THE BACK FOOT IS NOT ROLLED BUT PUSHED

Both the front foot and back foot must work together in doing this key. Because of this the back foot must also be moved in a relaxed and natural manner. Consequently, the back foot will roll gradually. If the back foot pushes instead of rolling gradually, usually the effect is too strong in that it will cause pressure on the hip of the back leg and the back foot becomes too dominant *(Illustration 95)*.

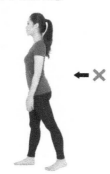

*Illustration 95: Back leg and back foot are pushed: pelvis of the back leg receives pressure, and the back leg will be too dominant*

## 2. THE BODY IS TOO FAR FORWARD BEYOND THE FRONT FOOT

If the body is too far forward to the point it passes the front foot, the pressure on the hips and front leg will be excessive. In this condition, the adjustments and natural changes on the body will not be able to happen well *(Illustration 96)*.

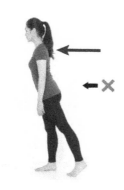

*Illustration 96: Body is too far forward beyond the front foot*

## 3. BACK LEG NOT SUPPORTING THE BODY

If **Key 3** has been completed and the back leg does not support the body, the muscles of the back leg are not used, and the body weight will all fall on the front leg. Consequently, the natural adjustments and changes will not be able to happen well *(Illustration 97)*.

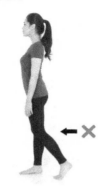

*Illustration 97:*
*Back leg not*
*supporting the body*

## 4. LOOKING DOWNWARDS

During the duration of **Key 3** or following it, do not look downwards. Let your view continue to be directed straight forward while being relaxed, because that is the most natural. If you are looking downwards *(see Illustration 98)*, the adjustments and natural changes will not be able to happen well. By looking downwards, not only will your neck be bent blocking the natural adjustments process but the various muscles in the body will also be tense, even to the sole of your feet.

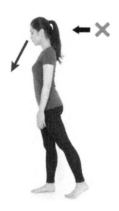

*Illustration 98:*
*Looking downwards*

## 5. BODY WEIGHT IS NOT EVENLY DISTRIBUTED ON THE FRONT FOOT

The importance for our body weight to fall evenly over the sole of the foot has been discussed a number of times. Our body weight must always be sufficiently and evenly spread over the outer, inner, front and back of the sole of the foot touching the ground. If our body weight is not spread evenly over the sole of the foot, our body will tend to sway and be unstable *(see **Illustration 99**)*.

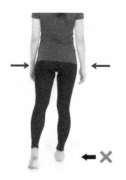

*llustration 99: Body weight not evenly spread over the sole of the foot*

# Chapter 15
## Key 4: Letting All Adjustments Happen

As previously noted, there is no movement in this **Key 4**. Rather, we intentionally do not move for a moment to give the time for the changes to happen in the best way possible on the whole body and its systems. Because there is no movement, the body position is still exactly the same as in the previous **Key 3**.

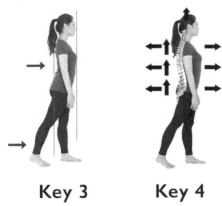

Key 3          Key 4

*Illustration 100: Key 4: Letting All Adjustments Happen*

## INSTRUCTIONS

- Stop everything.
- Let go of everything to let the natural adjustments happen starting from the soles of your feet, both feet, whole legs, whole torso, neck, each limb, your head, at the same time starting from the end of the tailbone moving upwards disc by disc while spreading to all directions. Also on each meridian and each reflexology zones, improving, rejuvenating, activating, reactivating and refreshing all systems and body organs to be the way everything is supposed to be until it flows through the crown chakra.
- Feel your breathing become much freer, your whole body becoming fresher, healthier and improved in every way.

## EXPLANATION

Why does the initial instruction of this key start with stopping everything? Because, although our body may have stopped moving, we are actually still getting ready to move our legs and body for the next step. Because of this, we must be reminded to stop completely. And for the best results, we need to be reminded again to let go of everything. Let the natural adjustments happen in the best way possible.

In our daily life, allowing the adjustments to happen on us is extremely rare and is something we possibly have never done before. This is quite logical, because people seldom understand that each step is a facility for the body to repair itself.

Other than this, most of us tend to often be in a rush in stepping to reach the desired destination. Stopping in each step to allow the natural adjustments to happen is not a common occurrence, even in the moments of extreme relaxation. Even if it is being done, the natural adjustments cannot happen without applying the SONW method. These natural adjustments will happen if we stop in each step. However, you may be surprised and confused. How would you be able to walk in your everyday life, in the markets, at the mall and so on? Do not worry, after gaining a proper understanding of this SONW method, you will be able to perform **Key 4** for a duration of only one second or less in each of your day-to-day steps. Although the adjustments will be rather limited, if you are doing it in every step, which may add up to thousands in each day, this will still provide benefits that are meaningful. However, if you do have special time to commit and wish to obtain the best results, perform **Key 4** as well as possible. Let the adjustments happen for a few minutes in each step. By doing this, you will be able to obtain tangible results in a relatively short period of time.

## BODY WEIGHT

The body weight, both in relation to the front and back legs and the left and right legs, is still exactly the same as on completion of **Key 3**.

## COMMON MISTAKES:

1. The stomach is pushed forwards
2. Adjusting the spine/body on your own
3. Some parts of the leg/body are lazy

To help you better understand, an explanation is given in relation to each one of these mistakes below.

## 1. THE STOMACH IS PUSHED FORWARDS

Whilst letting the adjustments happen, some people may start to feel the adjustments happening on their muscles, muscle fibres, meridians and so on in their legs all the way to the upper parts of the body. Feeling this, some may try to "help" the process of adjustment for this body part and end up pushing the stomach forward or pulling the chest *(Illustration 101)*. The best way is to just allow everything to happen naturally.

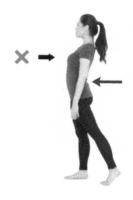

*Illustration 101: Stomach pushed out or protruding forward*

## 2. ADJUSTING THE SPINE/BODY ON YOUR OWN

Similar to the above, the natural adjustments should happen on the whole body including the stomach, chest, spine and even to the hands, fingers, neck and head. Everything has to be allowed to happen naturally for the best result. However, on feeling the natural adjustments happening some people try to help by providing an additional push to the spine or their own body *(Illustration 102)*.

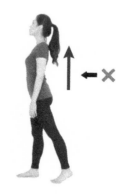

*Illustration 102: Adjusting the spine or body on your own*

## 3. SOME PARTS OF THE LEG/BODY ARE LAZY

This mistake is the reverse of the previous two mistakes. Whilst in the previous two mistakes the issue is that the person is too eager to help the adjustment process that is happening, this mistake usually happens because the person is "lazy". People who are "lazy" usually allow their knees, hips, stomach and various other body parts to "fall". In this condition, the natural adjustments cannot happen because it is being blocked by those "lazy" parts. The natural adjustments can only happen through the parts of the legs, hips, stomach and so on that are not lazy.

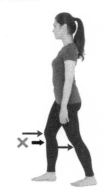

*Illustration 103:*
*Lazy part of the*
*body (knees)*

# Chapter 16
## Key 5: Letting Go of the Body Weight into the Earth

Key 5 is similar to **Key 4** in that there is no movement at all. The aim of **Key 5** is to let go of the body weight into the earth so that the body weight may reach the earth evenly. This allows the sole of our feet to step in an even manner, between the outer, inner, front and back parts *(Illustration 104)*. Our body position will also remain exactly the same as when we completed **Key 3**.

### INSTRUCTIONS
Let go the weight of your body through the front foot into the earth.

### EXPLANATION
By letting go of the body weight into the earth, we will become more relaxed. Many people in their daily life hold their body weight and become tense without realising it. Letting go of the body weight into the earth also helps in correcting the body posture. Although **Key 5** appears rather

simple and is rarely performed, this key is actually tremendously important. Only by performing this key properly will we be able to walk better and be more relaxed in our everyday lives.

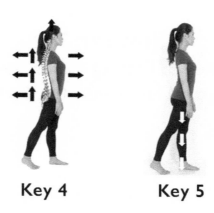

## Key 4          Key 5

*Illustration 104: Key 5: Letting Go of the Body Weight Into the Earth*

## BODY WEIGHT
Because there has not been any movement at all, the body weight is still in the same position as the point in time **Key 3** was completed.

## COMMON MISTAKES:
1. Not letting go the body weight into the earth
2. Letting go the body weight sideways

The following describes two of the common mistakes usually made in performing **Key 5**.

## 1. NOT LETTING GO THE BODY WEIGHT INTO THE EARTH

Sometimes, because of a habit of not letting go of the weight of the leg, or perhaps because this is seen as something trivial, the body weight is not released into the earth *(Illustration 105)*. Without letting go of the body weight into the earth, the hips will sway considerably when the next step is taken.

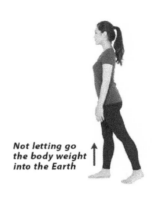

*Not letting go the body weight into the Earth* ↑

*Illustration 105: Body weight not released into the earth*

## 2. LETTING GO THE BODY WEIGHT SIDEWAYS

Because we often walk improperly, our body weight is not evenly supported by the soles of our feet. There are some people whose body weight falls more on the inner, back, outer, front or some kind of combination of the sole of the foot. If this happens, when letting go of the body weight into the earth there will be a tendency for the body weight to remain supported by the body or legs *(Illustration 106)* when it should be released naturally into the earth.

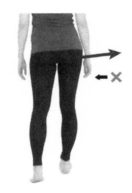

*Illustration 106: Body weight released to the side*

# Chapter 17
## Key 6: The Next Step

Key 6 is essentially the same as **Key 1**, with the exception that it is being performed by the other leg. Other than that, because the position of the leg to be swung forward will not be side-by-side as it is in **Key 1**, the back leg will first need to be relaxed to the point that the knee bends. At this moment the position of the leg will still be behind the other leg. Subsequently the leg is then swung forward exactly in the same manner as in **Key 1** *(Illustration 107).*

### INSTRUCTIONS
- Relax your back foot to rest on your toes with your knee folded
- with your whole leg directed straight forwards and your knee still folded, bring your back foot forwards as the next step

### EXPLANATION
If someone is able to perform **Key 1**, **Key 6** which is essentially the same as **Key 1**, will also be able to be

performed with relative ease. The most important matter to be remembered is that the back leg must be relaxed to the point that the knee is bent. If this is not done properly the back leg will still be touching the ground when being swung forward. The leg still touching the ground will have to be forcibly pulled in or outwards forming a curve to reduce the friction against the ground.

## BODY WEIGHT

Because **Key 6** is essentially the same as **Key 1**, the body weight being supported in between the front foot and back foot and between the left foot and right foot is exactly the same as in **Key 1** *(Illustration 108)*.

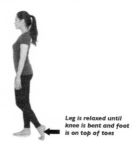

**Leg is relaxed until knee is bent and foot is on top of toes**

*Illustration 107: Swinging the back leg forward*

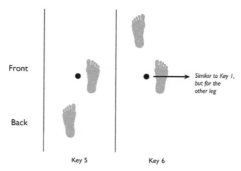

*Illustration 108: Shifting of the body weight between the front foot and back foot before and after Key 6: The Next Step*

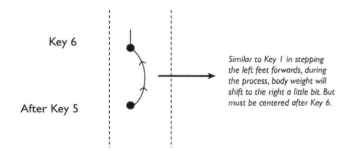

Key 6

After Key 5

Similar to Key 1 in stepping the left feet forwards, during the process, body weight will shift to the right a little bit. But must be centered after Key 6.

*Illustration 109: Shifting of body weight between the left foot and right foot before and after Key 6: The Next Step*

## COMMON MISTAKES:

The common mistakes in **Key 6** are:

1. Dragging the foot forwards *(Illustration 110).*
2. Curving the foot outwards *(Illustration 111).*
3. Curving the foot inwards *(Illustration 112).*

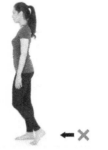

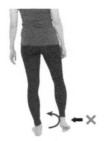

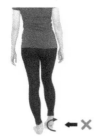

*Illustration 110: Dragging the foot forward*

*Illustration 111: Curving the foot ourwards*

*Illustration 112: Curving the foot inwards*

Practically, the common mistakes in performing this key are a combination of the common mistakes in **Key 1**, plus the three abovementioned mistakes. However, because it has been discussed in **Key 1**, it will not be repeated here. Meanwhile, for the three mistakes noted above, the cause is usually the same, that is the back leg is not sufficiently relaxed or the knee of the back leg is not sufficiently bent before the leg is swung forward. Because of this I have not separately discussed the issues in relation to these three common mistakes.

# Chapter 18
## Important Matters Related to Secrets of Natural Walking® (SONW)

### CHANGES TAKE TIME

In practicing the SONW method, some of you may start to realise how the way you had previously been walking is extremely poor. For example, the position of the soles of your feet are open or you pull your hips forward. It is vitally important to correct these mistakes. However, it is also important for you to remember that the muscles of your legs and body had been used in an improper manner for many years, or even decades. Do not force immediate changes, because it will result in pain or discomfort for your legs and/ or body.

### PEOPLE WHO FIND IT CHALLENGING TO PRACTICE SONW

If at this moment you are experiencing problems with your legs, hips or spine and wish to try to practice the SONW method, perhaps you may not be able to practice in the same manner as someone who does not have these ailments. For example, if you are experiencing difficulties in moving your leg or taking steps, or otherwise experience pain in doing so, it is recommended that you first practice **Key 1** and **Key 2** properly. Do it repeatedly around 20 to 50 times every time you practice (depending upon your ability to do it without forcing yourself). After practicing these two keys repeatedly for a week or more, usually there will be a clear improvement. For some people who are experiencing hip pain, the pain should disappear completely. After the problem or pain has reduced in intensity, the best is to perform all six steps of SONW consecutively.

## PEOPLE WHO REQUIRE A WALKING STICK OR OTHER WALKING AIDS TO ASSIST IN WALKING

For those people who require a walking stick or other walking aids to be able to walk, they may wish to hold onto something sturdy. The best is for the walking aid to be positioned beside the body, not in front. The walking aide should also be vertical, not horizontal because this will affect the placement of the body weight and the muscles that will be utilised. Specialised walking aids to support the body weight and other special aids are usually provided in the SONW practice places which are referred to as Walking Centers (further information provided in **Chapter 22**).

In practicing, one may hold onto these walking aids continuously, even whilst moving the legs. However, at the end of each movement, it is extremely important to let go of the body weight from the walking aids, even though one may still be holding it just to maintain balance. The body weight must be properly released into the earth to obtain the best results.

## SORENESS VS PAIN AND CLEANSING IN SONW

If you have attempted to practice SONW, you would have felt how the muscles of your legs, buttocks and various other body parts have become quite sore. This happens not only to people who seldom exercise, but also to people who routinely and intensely exercise. With SONW many muscles that are never or rarely used will be used and of course it will feel sore. This is actually something positive.

However, even though you may feel sore, you should not feel pain. If you feel pain, it is usually because you are not doing the SONW movements properly. Remember that SONW is a natural method to remind us to use our body naturally, that is not to force and control the body. If in practicing SONW you control or force your body, like pushing or throwing your heel when performing **Key 1**, you will feel pain in the related parts. So, if you feel pain, it is recommended that you consult with a certified and experienced SONW instructor.

Notwithstanding the above and as an exception, sometimes someone may feel pain in their shoulders, neck or surrounding area. As you are aware, the SONW method does not involve any other part of the body except for the lower parts. Usually if pain is experienced in the upper parts of the body, it is something positive. It means the adjustments, changes and reparations have reached the upper parts of the body. The chronic problems that exist in those parts are being healed and sometimes the process causes pain.

There are also people who when practicing SONW get swollen hands to the point that their fingers swell and turn reddish, blackish or even bluish. Similar to the previous explanation, in implementing the SONW method, you do not need to do anything directly to the upper half of the body, including the hands and fingers. The swelling of the fingers is good because it shows that the cleansing is happening to the upper parts of the body and the negativities are being pushed out through the fingers.

To accelerate and expedite the cleansing process, accompany your efforts with gratitude and prayer to our Creator. By being grateful, the process will happen more completely, and the best results may be had.

## SERIOUSLY VS CAREFULLY

To obtain the best results, you must practice seriously. Seriously means every day you must practice for a duration of one hour to one and a half hours. However, this cannot be forced. As previously discussed, if you have problems or otherwise are not strong enough to do it, do not force yourself. If it is possible, repeat it again after resting. However, if not, practice to the best of your ability routinely every day while slowly increasing the duration. Although practicing seriously is important, you must also do so carefully.

## OLDER PEOPLE IN PRACTICING SONW

If you pay attention, you will observe that older people usually walk with both knees slightly bent. Consequently, automatically the body will lean forward to compensate. When practicing SONW they will also tend to bend their knees. The problem is that whilst the knees are bent the natural adjustments will not be able to happen properly. Because of this, after such older people can start to be able to perform SONW well (after practicing routinely for around two to three weeks), they will need to be reminded to start to try to straighten their knees when practicing. Remember again that changes require time. So, do not ask them to straighten their knees on the first few days of practicing SONW. Also, do not force them to straighten their knees perfectly.

## SONW IS NOTHING SPECIAL

In this book I indeed have on multiple occasions stated how many people have obtained extraordinary results from practicing the SONW method. However, it is important for me to remind you how in my view this SONW method is actually nothing special. The SONW method does not have the ability to heal or help in any problems at all. You may be confused and start to wonder why I am going around in circles.

What I have expressed is important to be realised. The SONW method is only to remind us to start to use our body (in this matter, walking) as we should be (naturally). By using our body naturally, the extraordinary abilities within our body will be able to function again. So, what we must realise is that it is actually our body that has the extraordinary healing abilities. Our body is an incredibly beautiful gift of love from our Creator who loves and cares for us completely and always gives us the best.

Only by realising this will we be able to be even more grateful to our Creator. Why have I stated this? If you feel as a human who is extremely grateful to our Creator but decide to still walk in accordance to your old habits, it means you are still prioritising your own self-interest as opposed to your body. How can you claim to be extremely grateful to our Creator if the body given as a gift of love from our Creator is considered unimportant? Shouldn't that feeling of gratitude be expressed through actions?

## EXPRESSION OF GRATITUDE TO OUR CREATOR

If you have realised what I have discussed previously, the most beautiful is if in practicing the SONW method diligently and correcting the way you walk is no longer motivated for your health or even any of your priorities at all. Doing it all just as an expression of gratitude to our Creator. If you do this, you will be able to feel how you are more joyful in practicing SONW. Further, the benefits that will be obtained will be even greater. You will also start to be able to change your daily habits not only in walking, but also in various other aspects too.

As I have previously explained, if we are really grateful to our Creator for the gifts of love, we would certainly express these feelings of gratitude through our actions. We will definitely use our body better, including walking properly and also taking care of our body as best as possible.

As a note, you must do all of this wholeheartedly. Although we are familiar with the expressions "wholeheartedly", "bottom of my heart", "carefully" and "inner heart", in practice not many people do actually use their heart. As an example, understanding the importance of taking care of the cleanliness and health of our teeth does not automatically make us brush our teeth routinely, right? It is the same with the heart. Knowing that we must open and use our heart does not mean that we have actually used our heart. We must open our heart in the correct way. Information in relation to opening and using the heart may be read in the book *Smile to Your Heart Meditation: Simple Practices for Peace, Health and Spiritual Growth* that I have written several years ago.

## TAKING CARE OF OUR BODY AS BEST AS POSSIBLE

Implementing the SONW method does assist in stopping the various poor habits that we have been doing to our body for many years. The SONW method also restores the various natural abilities that has been granted by our Creator. However, just implementing the SONW method on its own is not enough. We also must take care of our body as best as possible in all other aspects. Especially, this also forms our real actions in expressing our gratitude to our Creator.

A few of the most important general aspects that we must do when taking care of our body include:

1.  Consuming healthy food.
2.  Sufficient rest/sleep,
3.  Sufficient exercise,
4.  Maintaining the body's cleanliness.

# Chapter 19
## Walking Naturally in Daily Life

After understanding how important and beneficial it is to be walking naturally in accordance with the SONW method, it is particularly important to walk as naturally and as often as possible. This is not only to obtain the various benefits for our health but also to prevent us from further harming our body. We can do it by using our body naturally in daily life, including while walking.

Indeed, the six basic keys of SONW, especially **Key 4**, show that we need to set aside a dedicated time and place to take each step. Although we must give enough time for **Key 4** to work, in our daily life it is impossible for us to walk while applying **Key 4** in every step.

Thus, for the best result in our daily life we need to do both:

- Purposely allocate time from 1 up to 1.5 hours every day to apply the complete SONW practice including **Key 4** to allow the changes in our body and health to happen as best as possible. Some people may wonder, do we really need to practice that long every day?

What if we only practice for 30 minutes? If someone practices for 30 minutes every day, he or she will obtain some benefits but usually these benefits will be rather limited. Changes that take place in the deeper parts usually happen after 30 minutes and best after 1 hour of practice. Certainly, for people who do not have time, practicing for 30 minutes is still better than not practicing at all. Those who cannot stand up and practice for 1.5 hours continuously can do it in several phases. It is recommended to divide into a maximum of three phases, that is three times 30 minutes for each phase.

- Slowly try to improve the way we walk so that every step in our daily life is a natural step in accordance with the six SONW key steps, except for **Key 4**.

Essentially, it is important to recognise your habits in your daily walking, and to let go of negative habits while starting positive ones. When you first start changing the way you walk to be in accordance with the six key steps of SONW, you may experience some initial difficulties. Remember that our habit is to rush, control or hold our body, etc. Walking daily in accordance with the six key steps of SONW, especially in public places, will feel strange. However, if you remember to keep doing it over and over again, eventually the way you walk in your daily life will improve.

Changing the way we walk in our daily life is very important. It is true that if you do not change the way you walk in your daily life, but you do 1 to 2 hours of SONW practice per day, you will still indeed obtain benefits. However, you will not obtain maximum results because your steps in daily life are still incorrect. Improper walking throughout your day will lessen the benefits from your SONW practice.

In relation to day to day life, many people have also asked the following questions:

- How do we run?
- How do we walk uphill or downhill on uneven and steep surfaces?
- How do we walk up the stairs?
- How do we walk down the stairs?
- How do we walk backwards?

## HOW DO WE RUN?

Running is very different from walking. Although there are positive benefits from running, there are also some side effects. Based on the results of various research, when a person runs, the pressure on their knees is very high every time the sole of the feet touches the ground.

In relation to SONW, when running it is best to ensure that the pads of the feet always lands on the ground to reduce the jarring motion on the knees, hips and the whole body.

## HOW DO WE WALK UPHILL AND DOWNHILL ON UNEVEN AND STEEP SURFACES?

If you walk according to SONW method, the way you walk would already be the best in relation to walking uphill and downhill on uneven or even steep surfaces. By walking according to the SONW method, automatically your 'grip' to surfaces will be stronger than usual. You won't slip easily and in addition you would be able to breath better and deeper.

## CLIMBING UP THE STAIRS PROPERLY

Similar to SONW, in climbing up the stairs, if the step is wide enough to accommodate the whole foot, place your heel on the step first, followed by the pumping the pad of your foot.

You need to have the key understanding of a common mistake, namely, rushing. Oftentimes, even when the knees and waist are still bent, the person has already swung the other leg to climb the next flight *(Illustration 113)*. For the best results, allow the knees, hips and the whole body to be straight first before taking the next step *(Illustration 114)*.

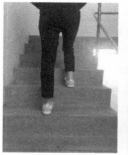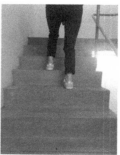

*Illustration 113: The improper way of climbing up the steps*

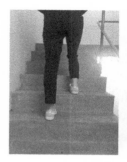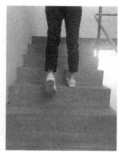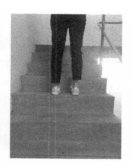

*Illustration 114: The proper way of climbing up the stairs*

## CLIMBING DOWN THE STAIRS PROPERLY

One common mistake in climbing down the stairs is: the back knee is not bent when stepping down, causing a strong impact, not only on the knee but also on the whole body.

In going downstairs, it is important to place the pad of the foot first. After the pad of the foot is in place, lower the heel. Only by first stepping with the pad of the foot can the impact from our body weight hitting the step be dampened. In addition to landing with the pad of the foot first, ensure that the knee of the back leg is bent a little to take on some of the body weight, thus dampening even further the impact of the body weight hitting the step *(see **Illustration 116**).*

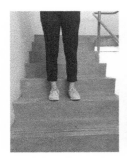
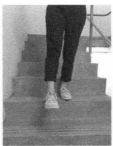
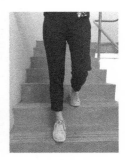

*Illustration 115: The improper way of climbing down the stairs: back knee is not bent*

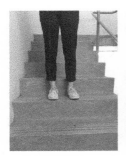
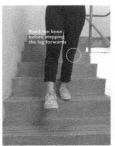
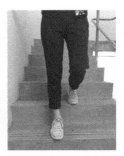

*Illustration 116: The proper way to climb down the stairs: bend the back knee before bringing down the front foot to land on the pad, followed by the heel*

## HOW DO WE WALK BACKWARDS?

To some of you, this question may be rather strange. However, in reality many people from all over the world have asked me this question. In relation to this question, I usually answer: our body is created by our Creator to be used to walk forward. If you have a hobby of walking backwards, please do not do it too often because it can cause negative effects on your body and overall health.

# Chapter 20
## The Discovery of Secrets
## of Natural Walking®

Matters related to the discovery of SONW is one of the topics commonly asked by many people. Where did the SONW method originate from? Because of that I will briefly share the background to the discovery of SONW in this chapter.

## BACKGROUND

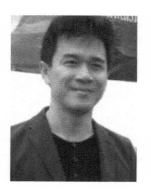

SONW was discovered by myself. The discovery of SONW actually started when I started to notice how the way my children walked changed with the different type of footwear worn, especially if the soles of the shoes were different from the previous ones. Interestingly, it was not simply the way they walked that changed. Just within several weeks, the shape of their legs also started to change causing their left and right legs to be imbalanced. They ended up being more emotional, more stressed, and so on.

By contrast, when they switched their shoes back and started walking better again, the shapes of their legs improved, their legs became more balanced and their calves became more toned. They also became more relaxed and smiled more. After years of observing this, I started to become certain that these were all related.

For those of you who have read my other books related to the heart and spirituality, you are aware that I often hold workshops in many cities in various countries. Therefore, I am acquainted with many people who often discuss new things that were realised through their hearts. I invited those people to observe together the connection between the way people walk with their leg shape, body shape, health, emotion, and mood.

After experimenting many times with many people from various cities and countries for several years, I summarised all of these experiments and saw the connection even clearer. It turned out that each of our steps indeed affected the shape our legs and even our whole body, and it only takes a short amount of time for our spine, body posture, meridians, reflexology zones, self-healing capabilities in our whole body to change.

The shape of the calves, legs, hips, chest, and whole body of many people have clearly changed. Problems in joint areas such as the knees, hips, waist, spine and shoulder vanished, including amongst elderly people. Various problems or even illnesses related to the internal organs were also greatly reduced or completely healed. The stamina, vitality, and so on also totally changed. Many of these changes could be said to have been an impossibility from a medical perspective. However, they did really consistently happen for many people.

Through these experiments, my theory that each of our steps will affect the shape of our legs, shape of our body, body posture, meridians, reflexology zones, self-healing capabilities in our whole body was proven. Each time it is repeated, the result is always satisfying. In fact, those who kept on practicing diligently have obtained even better and astonishing results.

## FORMULATING SONW

When the experiments started with only a few people, it could be done in a simple way. For instance, at that time, the common distance between the left foot and right foot is as wide as our shoulders because this was the common stance for sports and many physical movements. Likewise, there was no participant who had one foot shorter than the other.

However, as many more people started joining in these experiments, they came in various sizes and shapes. For example, there were people whose shoulders were very wide, there were children, there were also people who had one foot shorter than the other. I started to see that the general guidelines could not be applied to everyone. Thus, just like the example of the distance between left foot and right foot, there were several issues:

- If the width of the shoulders were the benchmark, those with wide shoulders and small hips would end up with too wide of a distance between their left foot and right foot.
- If we used a number as the benchmark, the number could not possibly be used for everyone of all sizes and proportions.

After further observation, I recognized that the best distance between the left foot and right foot should not be the shoulder width or a certain average number, rather it should be the width of the hip bone of each person. This is logical since our legs are located within our hip bone and therefore the best measurement is to use the same distance as the width of that hip bone.

As I found that the appropriate benchmark for the distance between the left foot and right foot is the width of one's hip bone, it was also discovered that the ideal distance between front and back feet is half the distance of the length of the foot of each person. Meanwhile, for people with one foot shorter than the other, when the shorter leg steps forward, the distance taken should be shorter than the distance taken by the other foot. After obtaining this additional information and sharing it to those who joined the experiment, it turned out that everyone obtained an even better result.

## FORMAL WORKSHOPS

After I felt that I had gathered sufficient information to help those with various conditions and differing body shapes, I offered an SONW workshop in October 2013, as a trial prior to rolling out the formal workshops. In the first workshop trial, I was stunned by the results obtained by the participants, as follows:

- Almost all participants who had problems with bowel movements experienced an improved digestive system on the same day of the workshop or one or two days after the workshop.

- Almost all participants who had tension in their shoulders, nape of their necks and the surrounding areas experienced significant improvements

- A 76-year-old lady who was hunched and was often exhausted experienced more energy and had a straighter back after 3 days of practicing SONW.

- Most female participants who practiced daily for one week reported changes in the shapes and firmness of their breasts, including those who were 76 years old and above.

- One female doctor who suffered from chronic constipation for decades, after a few steps of SONW her peristaltic bowel movement and habit suddenly normalized until now.

## THE DEVELOPMENT OF SONW

I am extremely grateful to our Creator for the chance to share with others how our body is truly a beautiful gift of love. I certainly hope that this SONW method may be learned by as many people as possible. Not only to be more grateful to our Creator, but also for us to be healthier and to have an improved quality of life. This is also why I have offered special training programs to those who have repeated the workshop and have practiced long enough, so that they too are able to teach others in order for everyone to obtain the best results.

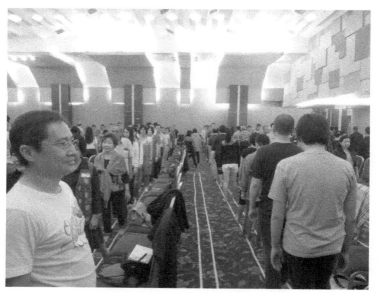

*Ilustration 117: SONW workshop in Jakarta, Indonesia*

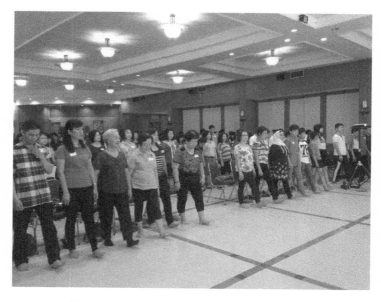

*Ilustration 118: SONW workshop in Medan, Indonesia*

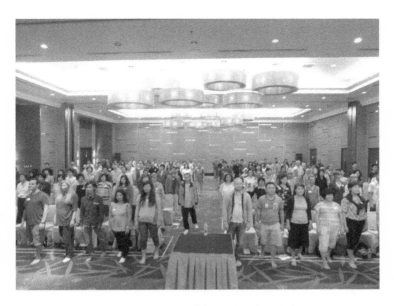

*Ilustration 119: SONW workshop in Bandung, Indonesia*

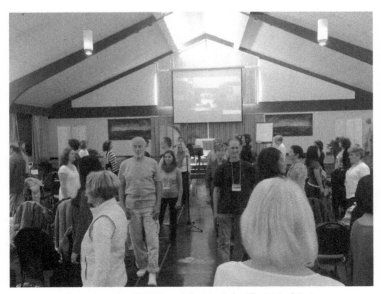

*Ilustration 120: SONW workshop in Asheville, United States*

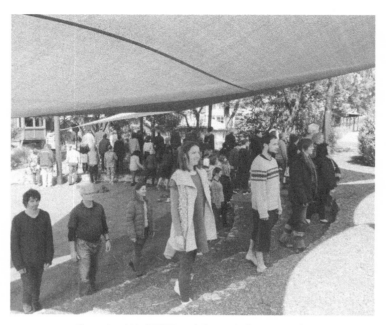

*Ilustration 121: SONW workshop in Hobart, Australia*

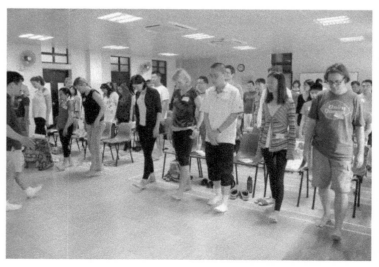

*Ilustration 122: SONW workshop in Hong Kong*

# Chapter 21
## Testimonials

The following are several additional testimonials from people who have recovered from various illnesses and problems after practicing SONW. Not only were their illnesses and problems healed, but the shape of their body, stamina, and function of their internal organs also clearly improved.

If you were to only read this testimonials section without reading the whole contents of this book, you might not believe these testimonials and may feel that these testimonials were made up. I hope that having read the details of SONW in previous chapters and reading real stories from real people in this chapter will help us all to realize better about our body being a special Gift of Love and to start using our body more according to the Creator's Will. May we express our gratitude to the Creator for the amazing capabilities that our physical body is equipped with by walking properly to maximize the wonderful, amazing natural functions of our body. Let us read some of the testimonials I have received from the various people who have practiced SONW over this time.

## No More Neck Tension;
## Rejuvenated and Energized

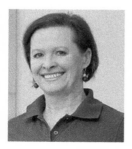

I am a physiotherapist who joined SONW in June 2015. Initially I didn't think that SONW would help me, but after I practice routinely, I realized how helpful SONW is. The tension on my neck disappeared, and I felt rejuvenated and energized. Secrets of Natural Walking® is a good and simple method to prevent many problems and can relieve existing health problems.

*—Heidi Zeschmann, Physiotherapist, Munich, Germany*

## The Disappearance of Back Pain

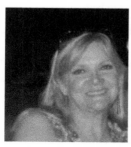

As a nurse anesthetist, one of the procedures I give is epidural steroid injections for people who are having back pain. This is done under live x-ray, and everyone in the OR must be protected by wearing heavy lead gowns and lead thyroid shields. This was giving me back pain! I told my husband I wasn't sure how much longer I could work, as I was in danger of becoming a pain patient myself. But after taking the SONW workshop and practicing at home, my back pain disappeared and I can keep working!

*—Dana Marino, CRNA, U.S.A.*

## Bye Sciatica! Hello Stamina!

Natural Walking is amazing. I am 64 years old and work 12-hour shifts as a Registered Nurse. I previously suffered from

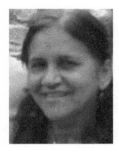

persistent sciatica and after a 12-hour shift at the hospital, I would be totally exhausted. My back and leg pain would escalate. As a result of Secrets of Natural Walking®, my sciatica is gone and my stamina and strength are beyond what I imagined I could ever feel at my age. I am able to work a 12-hour shift with a feeling of rejuvenation and joy. I encourage you to see for yourself what a transformative effect Secrets of Natural Walking® will have on improving all aspects of your life. Don't let life rush you by. Go for it!

*–Paramjit Rubenstein, RN, U.S.A.*

## Regaining Balance & Knee Improvement

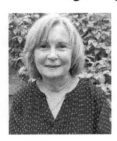

I was born with legs that curve inward, and I was told that when I was a baby, I wore leg braces. As I get older, whenever I got tired, my legs would bend again. As I got older, my knee would hurt, also because of a fall. After SONW, my knee no longer hurts.

I don't know of an official name for what ails my feet but an x-ray showed a bone spur. The podiatrist felt that was not the main source of problem, but instead might be arthritic gout. The doctor called it lymphedema of unknown origin and recommended physical therapy that would have cost

$2,000, so I didn't do it. I decided to just do Secrets of Natural Walking®. So much pain and swelling since last October is now down to 5% stiffness and swelling. I'm so grateful to have the use of my feet back! Walking in the sand at the shore at beginning of summer was not possible...but now it is...I'm so grateful and happy.

I broke my pelvis in 2002 when I fell from a bike...I already knew that I had osteoporosis as did my mother and I was just 55. After the fractures healed my one desire was to ride my bike again. After several attempts throughout the years, I still could not manage it due to balance problems I had since the fall. After two years of yoga, strength classes and balance, classes there was a little improvement but not enough to ride the old bike again. I stopped doing the yoga and other classes and have been doing the SONW regularly since May 2014. I was at my shore house in the beginning of July and there was the bike calling to me. I was a little scared but thought I'd give it a go.....it was so delightful to ride again and not one bit of balance trouble. I also can now climb up ladders to the top rung which I had been unable to do....

I am very grateful to the Creator for this most beautiful Gift of Love that is renewing us in so many ways...

Thank you, SONW.

**–Gloria Carroll, U.S.A.**


## Improvement in Neck and Shoulders

My experience with SONW has been quite unexpected. I have suffered from neck pain for years and the walking has helped to alleviate this pain. Since I began to take classes at the SONW Center I have experienced even more improvement to the point

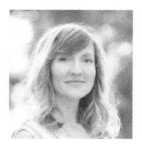

where the pain is almost entirely gone!

I am also standing straighter with my shoulders close to being level instead of one shoulder higher than the other. I can feel the physical changes happening ever-so-gently and I am thrilled to have more range of motion in my left shoulder and my neck again!

I highly recommend SONW and the SONW Center to anyone who is seeking to align body, mind and spirit and tap into their body's full potential. It's truly a transformative and enjoyable practice.

**–Krissy, Los Angeles, California, U.S.A.**

## No More Orthotics,
## No More Tension on My Right Side

Secrets of Natural Walking® is a simple yet amazingly effective

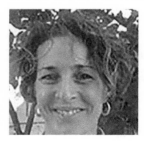

way of restoring your personal health and well being. As a former yoga teacher I practiced 3 hours a day for ten years trying to release tension and improve postural imbalances.

After attending my first SONW workshop, issues I had very consciously been attempting to fix for years were addressed. I no longer need to use orthotics, and the tension on my foot, neck, shoulder were released from the right side of my body.

As I continue to practice SONW I stand taller, have more

balance and muscle tone. I am emotionally lighter and more relaxed with my family, friends and colleagues. I no longer need to put effort into selecting asana postures and designing yoga asana routines. I simply enjoy the practice of walking naturally.

The most beautiful experience for me is to have found a practice that flows naturally into daily life. With each step, my body is being healed and my heart is being opened to Love, Life and all wonderful things from The Creator...

**–Jo Moloney, Alice Springs, Australia**

## No Longer Needing
## Special Insoles & Straighter Legs

I have had flat feet and had to wear insoles for the last 10 years,

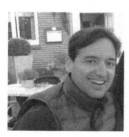

otherwise I would experience pain when walking. After diligent practice of Secrets of Natural Walking®, in only 2 weeks I no longer could wear the insoles as they became uncomfortable. So now I no longer wear any insoles ever! Also I was bow legged and notice my legs becoming more straight.

**–Patrick Rosalez, Los Angeles, California, U.S.A.**

## No More Stiffness

## on Foot from Plantar Fasciitis

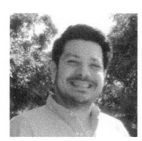

I've been struggling with stiffness in my foot from plantar fasciitis for the past year. After taking the SONW Bones and Joints class at SONW Center, the stiffness in my foot is no longer there and feels light and free.

−**Will, Los Angeles, California, U.S.A.**

## No More Incontinence;
## Overall Health Improvement

I had incontinence problem for a long time; I gave up running, dancing, and other types of sports. I did not even dare to run across the street. This was a big deal to me because I enjoyed working out. In 2011, I went to an incontinence specialist, and I was given various special

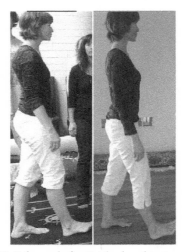

*Ilustration 123: Before and after Pat (neck and posture improvement)*

exercises to strengthen my pelvic muscles; however, after months of practicing, there was no improvement.

Everything changed after SONW: now, I am able to run downhill in my neighbourhood. I am very joyful and very grateful because not only was my incontinence taken care of, but I also experienced the following benefits:

✓ all my waist and back pain disappeared completely;
✓ my pelvic muscles became stronger;
✓ my shoulders/back straightened; I no longer slump;
✓ my whole body posture improves;
✓ I have better mood and am more joyful in my daily life;
✓ I am more energized, rejuvenated, and healthier.

—Pat, Australia

## No More Waist and Knee Pain

SONW has healed my 30-year chronic waist pain and 10-year chronic knee pain. Doctors told me that I just had to live with

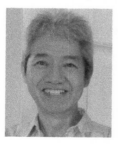

it, and for many years I took glucosamine/chondroitin, received acupuncture treatments, and sometimes did reflexology massages. Yet, none of those worked.

SONW, on the other hand, freed me from waist pain, knee pain, and now I am able to pick up heavy things without any pain whatsoever. At the age of 64, I no

longer feel old; I am now living life with a lean and proportional body.

—Willy Iskandar, Jakarta, Indonesia

## Many Benefits for 77-Year-Old Me

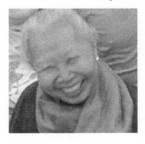

Because I was 77 years old when I first took SONW workshop, I did not expect much to happen on my old body. The many benefits I received from practicing SONW are: I no longer slump the way an old woman slumps; my back straightened, and I feel taller. Every muscle in my body is naturally lifted, and I am also stronger than before. Every part of my body feels more alive. I do not get sleepy as easily. My heart is calmer, and my mind is clearer. I enjoy practicing SONW very much, and I allocate time to do it every day.

**—Mrs. Iskandar, Yogyakarta, Indonesia**

### Benefits of SONW for an 85-Year-Old Woman

I am now 85 years old. About five years ago, I suffered from a collapsed disc in my spine due to degeneration, which caused a crack in the vertebrae. After being discharged from the hospital, I was still unable to sit up for long periods of time and had to rest lying on my back after sitting for 3-4 hours.

During the workshop, all the stiffness and pain from my back and entire body had gone and I felt fresh and relaxed immediately. I have been very diligent with my practice of Secrets of Natural Walking® and my daily routine of Secrets of Natural Walking® has helped me not only in strengthening my back, but my hunched back is now very much straightened too!

I suffered from the imbalance of fluid inside my ears, which

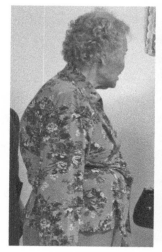
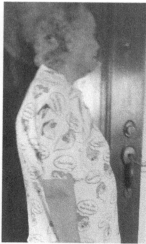

*Ilustration 124a: Before and After - Wung Hun Moi*

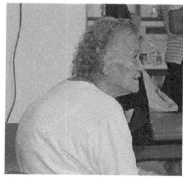
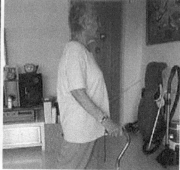

*Ilustration 124b: Before and After - Wung Hun Moi*

resulted in a loss of balance. However, one month into the practice of Secrets of Natural Walking® I was able to stand on the moving U-Shape machine for a good 5 minutes without holding on to anything. I also suffered from a mild stroke that resulted in the weakness and stiffness on the left side of my body - my left leg cannot bend at my left knee. For about 8 years, I had to lean on my right leg first when moving up or down the stairs and then lift my left leg to the same step before moving on to another step. I could not walk up or down the steps, placing only one foot on each step of the stairs. However, about three months into Secrets of Natural Walking®, I was surprised that I could bend my left knee while climbing the stairs! Now I can walk up or down the stairs with one foot on each step, and we believe that no medication or physiotherapy can give such amazing results!

Daily practice of Secrets of Natural Walking® has helped me very much for my whole well-being. I can bend my legs at my knees when walking up and down the stairs and my sleep quality has improved. Secrets of Natural Walking® has also helped me to keep a very calm disposition in many situations. My doctor complimented during one of my regular check-ups that I have maintained my general health above the average of old folks my age even after suffering from a mild stroke 8 years ago.

**–Wung Hun Moi, Singapore**

## Help for My Fibromyalgia

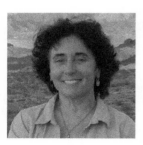

Incredible practice! I encourage everyone I know who has a desire to feel better, to try this workshop. It's helped me tremendously. No hip pain, no fibromyalgia pain, more toning, more energy, a calmer mind, and more peace-filled heart. Thank you to Diana for sharing her knowledge and gifts with me and many others!

**–Anita Adams, U.S.A.**

## Less Emotional and Straighter Back

I am a 76-year-old woman. Ever since I was 40 years old, my back already started to slump, and it became worse to the point where there was a hump on my back. With this condition, I found it difficult to walk far; I wasn't able to stand for too long because it would be painful; and even sitting or sleeping gave me pain. This caused me to be emotional.

When I was invited to attend SONW, I refused because I was sure that my back problem could not be healed because I was already old and this problem had been with me for 36 years and are getting worse by the day.

However, at the insistence of my husband and my daughter, I went to the workshop anyway.

During lunch break, I felt fresh, and after two weeks of practice, the pain in my back disappeared.

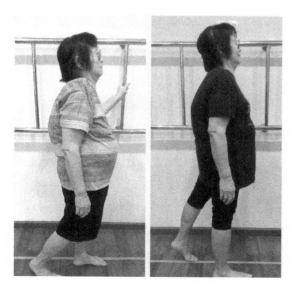

*Ilustration 125: Before and after - Agnes*

I stood straighter, and I could even run slowly (prior to SONW, it would cause me pain). My sleep quality also improved because I'm no longer in pain. My overall health improved tremendously.

To me, this is not about SONW, but about God's Blessings for me; a miracle. How could a health problem that had been plaguing me for decades be taken care of within several days!

My tip for everyone is: You must be diligent; don't be discouraged by tiredness when practicing SONW!

**–Agnes, Bandung, West Java, Indonesia**

### No More Insulin Injection + Increased Vitality

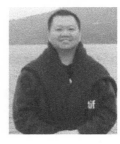

After my stroke at the age of 48, I needed twice-a-day insulin injection for my diabetes. Practicing SONW daily for week for 45 minutes each session lowered my blood sugar level. I amped up the 45-minute session to 1.5-hour sessions. My doctor told me that I could stop my insulin injection. SONW also made me leaner and healthier, and I feel fresh every day. My libido also increased.

**–Djohan, Jakarta, Indonesia**

## No More Back Strap/Back Support for Chronic Back Pain

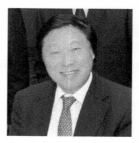

Secrets of Natural Walking® healed my back when everything else failed. I stopped using a back strap/back support, and I am now leaner; my mind is calmer; and my body is rejuvenated.

**–Murdaya Po, President of Indonesian Golf Association**

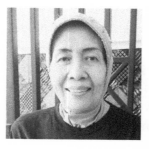

## Many "Miracles" through Secrets of Natural Walking

I am a retired 67-year-old medical doctor who attended Secrets of Natural Walking® workshop in January 2014, and I still practice SONW routinely up to now. I attended SONW with the curiosity to see if SONW could indeed resolve various health complaints. Having taken the workshops and having experienced what I call "many miracles" firsthand, I can say that SONW is quite logical and simple yet very effective and efficient in taking care of various health complaints with no adverse side effects.

- *4-cm height gain, 10-cm waistline reduction, 10-cm smaller hip size:* At the age of 67 and as a mother of 3 grown children, I gained 4 cm in height, lost 10 cm in my waist line, and lost 10 cm in hip size. When I was a young woman, I was slim, but aging had brought on consistent gain weight. It was after SONW that my body weight became stable at 45 kg, which is 5 kgs lighter than I was prior to SONW.

- ***Regaining right-knee functions***: I regained the functions of my right knee—it stopped functioning properly following a trauma when I was little.

- ***Reduction of joint and muscle pain:*** After SONW, the pain in my joints and muscles has lessened/completely disappeared.

- ***Re-growth of chest muscle 8 years after breast-cancer surgery:*** I had three major surgeries in my life: the removal of my ovary due to tennis-ball-sized myoma in 1993, right-breast surgery in 1994, and left-breast surgery in 2006 due to cancer. For the 2006 right-breast surgery, the cancer had spread onto my armpit, causing my right chest to concave after the surgery, making my left and right chest shape look imbalanced. After SONW, the shape of my right and left chest changed, making my left and right balanced.

With all of these amazing benefits SONW has given me, it was with gratitude to the Almighty and Most Loving Creator that I decided to become an SONW instructor so that I could share this natural method with fellow medical doctors, friends, and family members.

When I was still practicing medicine, I often met patients with health problems that required a lot of money to treat as well as a long period of treatment such as nerve problems, hernia, spine problems, stroke, diabetes, obesity, and many others that still ended up with residual problems or permanent disability. I also treated older patients with osteoporosis resulting in kyphosis or scoliosis along with organ damage because of their declining functions. After all that I have experienced with SONW, how could I not share this with others?

I invited fellow medical professionals to attend SONW workshop, and they were moved to suggest SONW to those who may benefit from SONW, and many of their patients have also reported wonderful, amazing healing. For example, we have had reports of trauma from accidents and surgeries being healed because of the perfect way the body is created by the Creator: simply by moving their bodies properly through walking, these patients allowed the meridians and reflexology points (which have been acknowledged by Western Medicine) to function simultaneously, speeding up the self-healing process.

I am very thankful to Irmansyah Effendi, the founder of SONW because he has helped me and so many others through this workshop. I hope many more people attend Secrets of Natural Walking® so that they too can be helped in their health problems.

**–dr. Nurlaita Hartono, Surabaya, East Java, Indonesia**

## The Return of Dislocated Disc to Its Normal Position

During an earthquake in Nias, an island near Sumatra, Indonesia, a big boulder from a building fell on me, popping

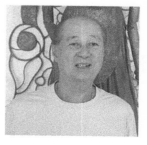

a disc on my spine out of its place to the point where the protrusion was visible. For one full year I had to wear a metal brace, and 8 years afterwards, I still could not lie down because my back still hurt. At SONW workshop, I could feel something happening on my spine, so I practiced routinely every day, and within three weeks, the disc returned to where it was supposed to be! I am now able to lie on my back and return to activities as if the accident never took place.

**–Yanto, Medan, Sumatra, Indonesia**

## Improvements on My Overall Health and Body Shape

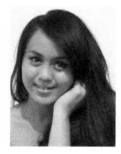

I had several health problems when I was little, and with typical additional activities as I grew older, I needed a fresh and fit body, but I didn't have that. I am still young (I am only 26 years old), and prior to SONW, for many years I was plagued with health problems that kept worsening. I was short of breath; I got exhausted easily, and whenever I was exhausted, I developed allergies and my endurance dropped; I had ulcer; my digestive system was bad (I had constipation), and so on. For years I had to deal with all these—I was constantly extremely uncomfortable, and to be honest, I was worried about my life.

On 12 April 2014, I attended Secrets of Natural Walking® with Irmansyah Effendi, and after practicing at home and repeating SONW workshops, my overall health improved. The pain in my body started disappearing; I now feel healthy and fit, allowing me to have more activities in life.

In addition to refreshing my body, SONW unexpectedly changed the shape of my body too: my hips that used to be wide and big are now more proportional; I no longer slump—I now stand straight effortlessly; and I feel very light. It feels amazing to not worry about my health and my life anymore.... (I don't know if the next one is connected to SONW or not, but after I became diligent in practicing SONW, money comes to me more easily)

**–Ida Ayu Putri Ciptasari, Bali, Indonesia**

### Rejuvenating

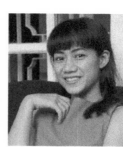

SONW was enlightening to me: I never thought much of walking, but SONW has helped me in my super-packed schedule to be fresher, fitter, and ready for the world.

**–Nia Dinata,**
Award-Winning Film Director, Jakarta, Indonesia

### Beating Anemia: Energy and Clarity

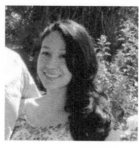

I've had Anemia for several years now and one of the symptoms is chronic fatigue and weakness. It was never a concern before since regular exercise and Reiki TUMMO self healings would help me manage the symptoms. However, 2-3 years ago it got really bad. I was falling asleep at 5-6pm and then I started feeling tired at 3pm and it became harder and harder to focus on conference calls and projects. It was like I had a cloud over me and my body could not function right - I could feel something was wrong. After an exam, my doctor shared that that my blood levels were dangerously low and that I needed an iron infusion immediately. I am very sensitive to medication and couldn't even take the iron supplements, so this really scared me. At the time, I really didn't have a choice so I decided to move forward with it. The treatment took place at a cancer hospital where people went in for chemotherapy. I had to go for 1-2 hrs/day for 10 days straight (+ I had to pay $1500; my insurance covered $2000). It was a lounge so everyone could see each other getting their treatment. I would get there, put on my headset and joyfully do my prayers.

I went in after one month and the doctor confirmed that my body had accepted the treatment (there was a chance it would reject it) and I felt better than ever for at least a year or so but then again slowly, I started to feel the fatigue despite my change in diet.

During the SONW workshops I could feel the energy flowing through my entire body and with practice I could feel the difference more and more clearly. I feel even better than when I received the treatment. There is a clarity that I haven't felt in a long time and my body feels alive - I don't feel like taking naps at all. I feel an improvement in my energy levels and my concentration levels at work.

Everything takes practice, though. The more I practice, the better I feel. I'm so grateful for SONW workshops and can't wait to start to share more with others.

**–Jennifer Plasencia, Los Angeles, California, U.S.A.**

## Beating Candida

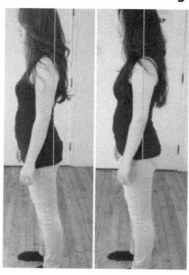

For the past 5 years, I had been having issues with my liver, suffered candida, and had lower back and neck pains. My eyes were constantly bloodshot red. People thought I was tired or stoned all the time. My candida was so bad that it broke out into my skin and had constant itching and eczema. It was so bad that I was unconsciously scratching while sleeping that I would wake up bleeding. I couldn't walk for more than an hour before: my back would be so sore and would have to sit down and rest. Sitting in front of the computer all day, every day, gave me lower back and neck pain. Driving home for the 1-hour commute and then standing in the kitchen to cook dinner was a real struggle.

My eye doctor suggested I get eye surgery and have plugs put in my eyes. My medical doctor diagnosed me with a skin disease. I just didn't believe them, so I sought alternative treatments and for 4 years saw acupuncturists, stayed on strict diets, and spent over $4,000. Unfortunately, the issues were never healed, but instead only managed. The last acupuncturist I saw diagnosed my liver as being damaged from all the antibiotics, birth control, alcohol, and processed foods I had eaten all of my life.

After taking the Secrets of Natural Walking® Workshop, I practiced every day for only 30 minutes to an hour a day. My diligence was surprising because I was never able to get into the habit of exercising regularly before. More than I've ever felt in years, I started feeling stronger and more energized.

The only thing I did was Natural Walking and after only 2 weeks, I could no longer walk the old way. After 6 weeks, my posture straightened and I felt taller. When walking up a flight of stairs, I no longer got winded. Even sitting at my desk all day, I felt no back or neck pain at all! Normally if I went shopping for over 2 hours straight, I would have lower back pain, but this time I actually felt more energized with each step. I no longer had pain and didn't need to take a break by sitting down. After measuring myself, I realized that I had lost 4 centimeters off my waist and hips, my left and right leg became the same size, and my breasts became fuller.

It has been 3 months since taking the workshop and I'm still practicing every day and loving it. My candida is gone, no itching, no eczema, and my eyes are clear. Old bumps/scars from the itching have disappeared. My posture has improved so much and my shoulders are straight now. Now I can have bread, sugars and some caffeine without any side effects. I am feeling healthier than I have ever felt in a very long time. My whole body feels stronger, so energized, and so much happier overall!

**–Anyez Cheung, Los Angeles, California, U.S.A.**


## Getting the Ideal Cholesterol Level
## in Half the Time

My cholesterol level was already not good even when I was still in medical school: my LDL (bad cholesterol) level was >120 mg/dl and my HDL (good cholesterol) level was only 20-30 mg/dl,

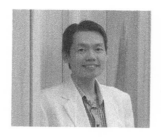

so I was told that I was at risk of getting heart disease. I had been meaning to improve my health, but being a medical student and later on as a medical doctor, my busy schedule made it challenging for me to eat properly or do physical exercise regularly. When I heard about Secrets of Natural Walking®, I thought, "Nice, I don't have to do intense workout; simply by mere walking I can be healthy, but is it really true??" Years of medical training made me skeptical—these are the things that should be questioned in the medical field. I did, however, remember that when I was studying Occupational Diseases, the medical field did claim that we can get sick from bad working habits; thus, I felt that there is logic to SONW's claim that improper walking can cause health problems. Based on this, I gave SONW workshop a try.

After one month of sporadic practice, I did not feel much change except muscle soreness. I did not expect SONW to improve my cholesterol level, so I was very surprised to see the lowering of my cholesterol level: my LDL became 102 mg/dl, and my HDL 46 mg/dl (though the risk of a heart disease was still at the 3.7 ratio). This test result motivated me, so I asked authorized SONW instructors to guide me further, and I joined group practices with fellow SONW workshop alumni so that I could practice more diligently.

The following two months, I practiced SONW diligently, and I attended the Health Retreat + SONW workshop taught by the founder of SONW, Irmansyah Effendi. The next blood-test result AMAZED me: I had an ideal cholesterol level! My LDL level was 96 mg/dl, and my HDL was 56 mg/dl, lowering my total cholesterol level by 161 mg/dl, and the risk of a heart disease drastically lowered to 2.9. As a medical doctor, this defied my medical knowledge: according to Gilbert R. Thompson, Emeritus Professor of Clinical Lipidology at Imperial College School of Medicine, it takes 4 hours per week of exercise in the course of 5 months to raise the HDL level by 5 mg/dl. Yet there I was with the significant improvement of my cholesterol level in a shorter time from doing Secrets of Natural Walking® practice.

**–dr. Julius Pangayoman, Bandung, West Java, Indonesia**

## The End of Chronic Leg Shrinkage and Re-Growth

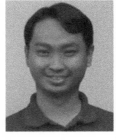

Decades ago in junior high school, I got into an accident resulting in broken bones and inflammation of the bones. Even up to recent years, very often the inflammation would flare up, and I also would get suppurative infections and inflammation. In addition, the hurt leg kept on shrinking to the point where it became 11 cm short er than the other leg. However, after practicing SONW, the hurt leg improved: I no longer experienced infection or inflammation. Also, SONW helped me gain 1.5 cm back: now that leg is 9.5 cm shorter instead of 11 cm shorter than the other leg!

**–dr. Noor Khalis, Bandung, West Java, Indonesia**

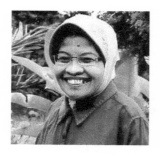

## Improved Eyesight and Scoliosis

I am very grateful to the Creator because through SONW practices, at the age of 61, my eyesight prescription went from -3.50 to -3.0 and within six months, it improved even further, becoming -2.2 and my astigmatism is totally gone.

SONW also improved my spine: my dextroscoliosis "straightened" without surgery, resulting in feeling light, more energized, and happier. I'm very grateful to Creator. May many more people be helped by Secrets of Natural Walking®.

**–Dr. Erna Karim, Jakarta, Indonesia**

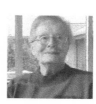

## Rheumatoid Arthritis

I attended my first session of the course (Secrets of Natural Walking) and at the end, found the pain in my shoulders had vanished and I could raise my arms above my head so easily and painlessly. Imagine my surprise on the next day to find I could stand up from the settee with no pain and no need to have someone haul me to my feet. This has continued to my amazement and delight!!

**– Bertha, Hobart, Australia**

## Kennedy Disease:
## No More Walking Cane, Younger and Healthier

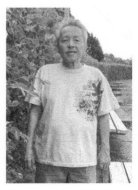

For 20 years, I suffered from "Kennedy" disease, which is a spinal bulbar muscular atrophy where my whole body even my tongue and voice box weakened. I had to use a cane to walk. According to my neurologist, there was no medicine nor solution for this. I also tried acupuncture, Chinese doctors, and other treatments, all to no avail. Gradually, my condition worsened.

After practicing SONW for three months, I experienced real improvements on my body: I did not need the walking cane anymore; I feel rejuvenated; and I have become healthier. Those who know me told me that I look younger than before I attended SONW workshop.

**–Bernard, Sydney, Australia**


## Hair Re-Growth on Bald Spots from Alopecia!

I was diagnosed with Alopecia, an autoimmune disease that causes me to have random bald spots on my head. I had to shave off my head to hide my condition, and I had to wear a hat everywhere I went. I lost my self esteem and was sad because I was not able to take off my hat in many events. I even got into a depression and lost enthusiasm in my job and social life.

I tried all kinds of treatments from western medicine to

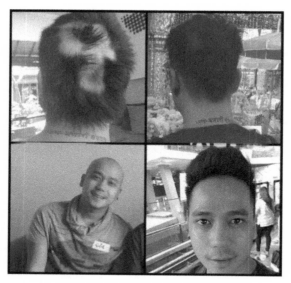

*Ilustration 126: Before and after: Gia's Alopecia improvement*

alternative healing, and even doctors said that it was very difficult to heal my disease and that it would take years of continuous treatment for my hair to grow again.

One day, without any hope, I attended Secrets of Natural Walking® workshop. It is true that after the workshop, I felt fresher and happier; I went from being stressed out to finding energy and renewed enthusiasm. Then I became lazy in practicing because I was busy and I wasn't motivated to do the practice by myself. After several months, my brother invited me (forced me) to participate in 21-Day SONW Challenge where we were expected to practice SONW for at least 60 minutes for 21 consecutive days.

On the second week of regular SONW practice, I went for my regular medical check-up, and my doctor was surprised to see several spots of new hair on my head! I was more surprised than my doctor, and I became more motivated to do SONW practices.

Even after 21 days, I continued doing SONW routinely, and I am happy to report that my hair is BACK!! Never in a million years would I ever think SONW could give me this extraordinary result!!

*—Gia, Yogyakarta, Indonesia*

### Priceless SONW

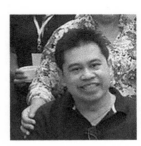

Thanks to SONW workshop, I went from spending $1,400 per month to a mere $20 per month on medication due to my stroke. That should give you an idea what type of improvement I got from SONW. I was shocked and very grateful. SONW is precious to me.

*—Unang Burhanuddin, Surabaya, East Java, Indonesia*

More testimonials can be found at:
*www.natural-walking.com*

# Chapter 22
## Additional Information

Although I have presented thorough information on Secrets of Natural Walking®, getting a direct guidance from an authorized SONW instructor at SONW workshops and SONW Center will expedite your improvements.

*www.natural-walking.com*

You can find information on worldwide SONW workshops and SONW instructors on www.natural-walking.com. SONW workshops are held regularly all around the world. Please find the nearest SONW Instructor in your area and register for his/her class. For urgent questions, please use:

**Whatsapp:** +62 877 8850 1144

In addition to the workshops, there is also support from SONW Center.

## SONW Centers

Practicing is very important as it helps:

✓ remove bad walking habits
✓ start natural-walking habits
✓ obtain results for overall health

At any SONW Center worldwide, you can practice walking naturally:

- ✓ under the direct guidance of fully-trained SONW instructors who can give you personal consultations
- ✓ with other SONW-workshop alumni to motivate you to practice more
- ✓ with better understanding and practical applications of the keys to obtain the best results
- ✓ with special exercises to help speed up the termination of bad habits and the improvements on certain body parts
- ✓ maximizing results/improvements on your physical body, mind, mood (the lessening of negative emotions and the strengthening of the beautiful feeling from your heart), and overall health.

## Classes at SONW Centers

SONW Centers offer targeted exercises not available at SONW workshops. Some SONW Centers offer the following classes: Vitality, Anti Aging, Bones and Joints, Body Shaping, Health and Happiness, and FitWalk.

### Social Media Presence
Facebook:
https://www.facebook.com/naturalwalking/

Instagram:
@naturalwalking
Instagram.com/naturalwalking/

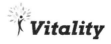 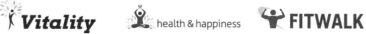 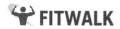

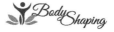 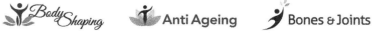 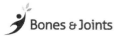

*Ilustration 123: Various programmes/special practices at SONW Centers*

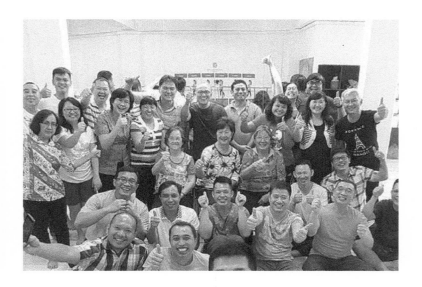

*Ilustration 127: SONW Center Jakarta, Ketapang*

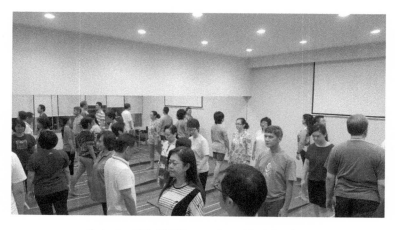

*Ilustration 128: SONW center Ivory Hotel, Bandung*

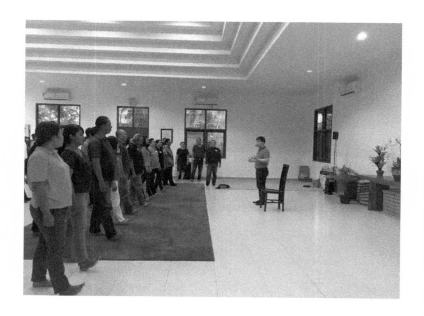

*Ilustration 129: SONW center BPH, Bali*

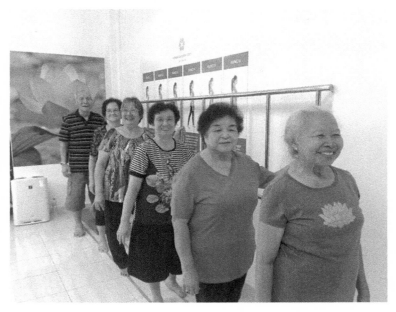

*Ilustration 130: Elderly practicing at SONW Center*

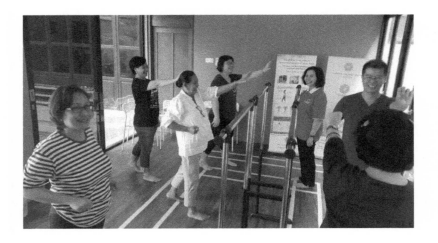

*Ilustration 131: SONW center, South Jakarta*

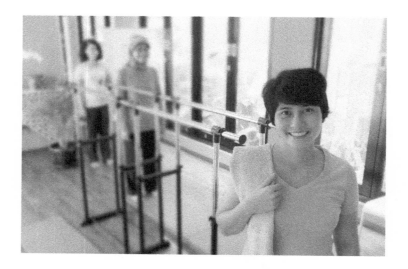

*Ilustration 132: SONW center, South Jakarta*

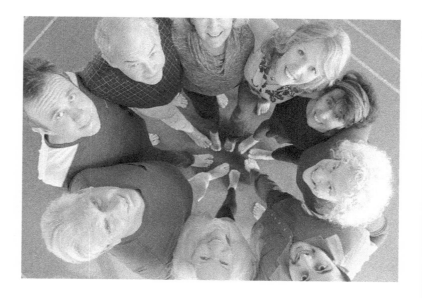

*Ilustration 133: SONW center, Asheville, United States*

# Works Cited

Cole. "How Old Is Your Body Really?" *npr.org*. June 28, 2016.
Web. 18 September 2016

"How Do All the Systems Work Together?"*slideshare.net*.
March 6, 2013. Web. 10 October 2016

Jockers. "Bad Posture Equals Bad Health."
*naturalnews.com*. Web. 10 September 2016

Mills and Square. "The Winsor Autopsies: Can an Unhealthy
Spine Affect Internal Organs?" Web. 10 August 2016

"Why Walking?" www.heart.org. Web. 6 August 2016

## Favourite SONW Instructors

### John Dunham, Canada

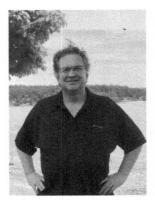

I was introduced to the Secrets of Natural Walking® in the spring of 2015, wondering at the time, "Why would anyone ever need to take a course on walking?" I have found out subsequently that is a very common reaction with most people, but I no longer ask myself that question. Through the Secrets of Natural Walking®, I have come to understand the importance of each step we take, and how each step can be a chance to reconnect with the earth.

We've evolved walking, and have walked as a species for millennia. Despite our long history with walking on the earth, most of us have no idea how important and beneficial our relationship with the earth can be. In the Secrets of Natural Walking®, you will learn how simple adjustments to your posture, and slight corrections to your steps will help you to be aware of your earth connection, and allow your body to let that connection do what it has been designed to do, and adjust our bodies to the way they are meant to be.

Ask yourself, "Are you aware of your connection to the earth with each step, are you feeling your connection to the earth with each step?" If not, let the Secrets of Natural Walking® help you to rediscover this wonderful gift.

Walking connects us with everyone else walking on the earth, and with everyone who has ever walked on the earth. That realization is more profound the more I come to understand it. If you are the least bit interested in sharing that understanding, contact me for workshop info, and you'll never have to ask again, "Why would anyone ever need to take a course on walking!"

I live on Salt Spring Island in the beautiful Gulf Islands of southwest British Columbia in Canada. I usually teach in the Victoria area, but with a little coaxing, and some interested students, I will gladly come to your community and share the Secrets of Natural Walking®.

Email:   jrdunham@natural-walking.com
             jrdunham@shaw.ca
Phone:  +1 (250) 537-4942 (Home)
             +1 (604) 837-4942 (Mobile)


**Dana Marino, Pennsylvania, U.S.A.**

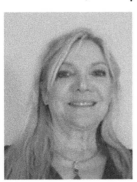

I live in Exton Pennsylvania in the western suburbs of Philadelphia. SONW has taken care of my lower back pain. And, amazingly, my height has increased by nearly an inch! We commonly shrink with age, and I had shrunk by an inch in height. But after the first 6 months of doing SONW regularly, my height was back to normal. A dear friend of mine got relief from chronic longstanding pain and fatigue due to Lyme disease after her first session! And it is so much improved over all! SONW seems to have wonderful anti-aging effects on the whole body. No one believes that I am almost 67 years of age.

Also, the calming, anti-anxiety effects are remarkable. It is truly like a miracle to me, and I am so grateful to True Source every day!

*Email: danacrna4@hotmail.com*
*Phone: 484-678-7721*

### Georgina Michael, Tasmania, Australia

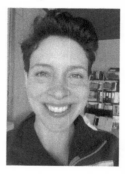

I never thought that my body was something beautiful to be compared to the wonders of nature. I always considered myself separate from the earth. SONW has demonstrated to me that as human beings we are so blessed beyond belief to have a physical body and that this body is so beyond any human biology textbook explanation I've ever read.

Practicing natural walking and surrendering the control of my body is awakening my being to the beauty of life, the special connection I share with the earth, and the simple sweet things in life that have been freely given. I grew up in a family where mental health is a major issue. I self-harmed through adolescence to the point of a suicide attempt. I hated myself and my body for many years, and food was a way to punish, control and soothe myself. I was so disconnected from my body in my first SONW workshop that I could not feel my body at all; I could only experience it by watching from a distance. The deep healing my being has gone through by allowing my body to walk naturally again has been so profound that it has changed my understanding of health and what it is to be 'healthy'.

Email: *georgy@happyswimmers.com.au*
Phone: *+61 410 247 346*
Facebook: *Secrets of Natural Walking Tasmania*
Facebook: *Lotus Centre Natural Walking*

## Geraldine Tobin, Ireland

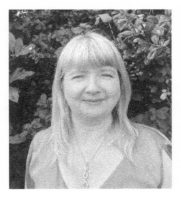

I would like to share how Secrets of Natural Walking® has had such a positive impact on my life and how wonderful it is to see the impact it has had on many others. I have EDS (Ehlers-Danlos syndrome) which is a collagen disorder. It can affect any organ, joint or tissue and any system like the circulatory system. It has quite a lot of symptoms but the most difficult symptoms for me have been joint pain and fatigue.

In April 2014, I went to my doctor as I had been waking up with the pain in my hip 3 or 4 times a night for over a year. My doctor told me all that could be done was a hip replacement, but she told me to try and wait for a few years (ironically, she told me to walk the pain out). So in May 2014, I attended my first SONW workshop. I was so bad: I had no balance; I couldn't straighten my back leg; I was completely out of alignment; and much more.

I practised daily and slowly my balance etc. began to improve. I had discomfort in my hip rather than pain. Later that summer, I attended Secrets of Natural Walking® Instructor Training. As I was practicing Natural Walking for a few hours during the day, I could really feel as an adjustment happened in my right hip which had the most pain: it would work its way up slowly so that my shoulder etc. would adjust.

This continued for months, and four years later it is continuing. But I never woke up again with pain from my hip and will not be getting my hip replaced. The important thing to know is that continuous practice will lead to continuous improvements. I have noticed that even if I stopped for a few days especially in the first year, I would have pain again.

The second thing is that it is a slow and steady improvement. I am still noticing improvements ...but it is amazing how much it has helped and continues to help.

Fatigue is another common symptom of EDS and I have found SONW fantastic for improving my energy levels too.

I am so grateful to have found this practice which has genuinely made such a huge difference to my quality of life. It is such a gentle, safe modality for everyone. I have taught Secrets of Natural Walking® to children from 6 years old to the more mature adults up to 80 years old and all have benefitted learning this lovely modality, especially those who enjoy Natural Walking daily.

*Phone: +353 874170764*
*Email: geraldine.naturalwalking@gmail.com*
*Web: www.naturalpath.ie*
*Facebook: SecretsofNaturalWalkingIreland*

**Laura Fan, U.S.A.**
Laura Fan teaches SONW in English, Mandarin, and Cantonese. Laura serves the following areas in U.S.: Walnut Creek & all San Francisco Bay Area, Sacramento (California,

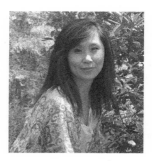

and Raleigh-Durham areas (North Carolina) Laura can also teach SONW in Hong Kong and Taiwan.

Secrets of Natural Walking® has brought about a total transformation for me from inside out. As a professional dancer and dance coach in the Dancesport industry, I was always exploring various modalities to enhance performance on all levels including body conditioning, fitness, and mental preparation.

After experiencing tremendous benefits from SONW in 2014 which helped heal my digestive system disorder, I decided to become a certified SONW instructor to share this beautiful and transformative modality for total well-being.

I am deeply grateful for the opportunity to be studying under the guidance of Master Irmansyah Effendi Msc. who who has patiently taught me how to approach life moment by moment through spiritual heart guidance.

I have since incorporated Master Irman's Open Heart and SONW in all of my dancing as well as teaching to help students manage competition or performance anxiety and at the same time improve their overall body awareness, coordination, balance, core strength and flexibility. I have also helped students to embrace SONW as part of their daily routine to improve their health conditions, including normalization of blood pressure, cholesterol level, anxiety management, and recovery from minor stroke.

*Email: LFan18@yahoo.com*
*Phone: +1 510 501-2925*
*Languages: English, Mandarin, Cantonese*

*Areas: New Jersey, Walnut Creek & all San Francisco Bay Area, Sacramento (California, U.S.A.)*
*Raleigh Durham areas, North Carolina, U.S.A.*
*Hong Kong*
*Taiwan*

### Cheynie Sukha, Tasmania, Australia

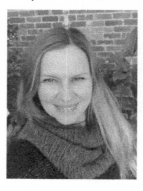

As an SONW instructor of 5 years, it never ceases to amaze me the changes that I witness in participants from the beginning of a one day workshop to the end. Participants of all ages physically perk up before my eyes, and lighten up emotionally once we begin the natural walking keys. The smiles and laughter follow and one can almost hear the sigh of relief the physical body breathes out, as much of the pressure and holding caused by unnatural walking is released. The changes are so sweet and obvious that I often take a before and after photo for participants to take home to inspire them to continue with their daily walking practices.

I am so grateful that we all have this chance to become more natural, more like how we were meant to be, and it feels like such an important gift that needs to be shared with everyone.

*Phone: +61433 324 534*
*Email: Cheynie@natural-walking.com*
*WhatsApp: +61433 324 534*
*Skype: Cheynie.sukha*

## Nikoletta Kovacs Kha, Melbourne, Australia and Hungary

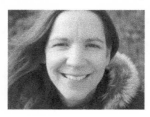

I have found SONW life-changing and happily see it improve the quality of life in many people around me.

*Phone: +61 437 550967*
*Email: nikikha@gmail.com*

## Amanda Young, Tasmania, Australia

Natural Walking has absolutely blown me away. The changes that can happen during this course and follow up practice are phenomenon. I feel like a new person after every workout. It not only changes your physical body but can change your whole attitude so you can be stress free, happy, without burdens even if things in your daily life are difficult. It is simple, yet deeply profound. It is easy for everyone to experience and share with each other. I teach Natural walking as it is one of those amazing gifts you are sometimes able to come across and when you do you just want to share it. I am truly grateful to have been able to witness the health and happiness in others because of this course.

*Email: amanda@lotuscentre.org*
*Phone: +61430282073*

## Donna, Melbourne, Australia

As a Fitness Professional and Master Trainer, I was very active with all types of intense physical exercise for over 20 years. As a result of training, I had acquired many injuries which resulted in continual consultancy with physical therapists and osteopaths to relieve pain. This therapy was incredibly expensive and painful, and I assumed that I would always have to continue managing the pain and injuries every 5 - 6 weeks as long as I was active.

I first heard about the physical and healing benefits of Secrets of Natural Walking® in 2013 and was curious to find out if it could help my injuries heal and eliminate pain.

The one-day course covered clear take home instructions on how to activate the body's natural healing ability and improve body shape, muscle tone and mental wellbeing. I practiced daily, and after 6 weeks I was pain-free. I also realised I had gained so much more: my posture had changed; I was standing taller; my leg muscles changed shape and were more in proportion with the rest of my body; and I also noticed the back of my legs were more toned. In addition to all those, there were noticeable mental and health benefits also. All the physical changes were quite surprising as I had been training myself and others very intensely in the gym 6 days per week for over 20 years.

It is possible to gain incredible results from walking properly using all the muscles of the body. I now include Secrets of Natural Walking® as a part of my daily training and have seen some incredible transformations in myself and others. I am now totally pain free; I have not seen a physical therapist since commencing the program in 2013. I highly recommend Secrets of Natural Walking® as a part of your daily routine to improve muscle tone, physical health and mental well-being and to eliminate pain.

*Donna Ellerton*
*Fitness Presenter, Master Trainer, Secrets of Natural Walking Instructor*

Phone: +61 479 063 285
Email: info@wellbodyandspirit.com
Instant Messaging/WhatsApp: +61405514462

## Narelle, Melbourne, Australia

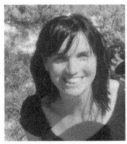

My first experience with the Secrets of Natural Walking *(SONW) was surprising and memorable. I felt deeply soothed to the core in a sweet and gentle way. It was fascinating to realise that the way I walked had been affecting not only my physical body, but also my mind and my whole being. As I continued to practice the walking my body started to change, old injuries started to heal, I slept well, my immune system improved and I enjoyed an increase in energy and vitality.

Naturally I felt to share this extraordinary practice and I began to teach. Over the years I have witnessed so many remarkable and miraculous changes in the workshop participants. As SONW activates the body's natural healing ability, it has been a gift and a relief for people managing injuries, mental health issues, stress etc. I have been very fortunate to witness the rapid and positive changes that have occurred in people, their bodies and in their wellbeing.

I'm very happy to be teaching and sharing this extraordinary and life changing practice. I invite you to join a workshop so that you can experience the wonder, peace, lightness, healing and vitality too.

Email: narelle@natural-walking.com
Phone/WhatsApp: +61 411607025

### Sunny Tjandrakesuma, Perth, Australia

SONW is awesome because after practicing it regularly my energy level is increased and also my immunity level, my whole being is more at peace and happy.

Please join the SONW workshop and reap all the beautiful benefits for your health and also your well-being in terms of feeling calm, happy and centred/grounded.

*Phone: +61438510671*
*Email: isk@iinet.net.au*

### Clare Jennings, Melbourne, Australia

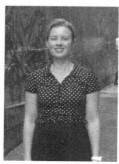

As you know we are so grateful to be able to offer you Natural Walking in your city. Natural Walking has brought me immense pleasure from walking more naturally and feeling more grounded to correcting my posture and helping me repair my pelvic floor muscles after having a baby. If you would like to experience all the benefits for yourself let us know.

*Phone: +61 409 385 792*
*Email: clare.jennings1@bigpond.com*
*Web: www.naturalwalking.com.au*

### Josephine Moloney, Alice Springs, Australia

The beauty of SONW is it supports physical, emotional, social and spiritual aspects of our health and wellbeing. It is an

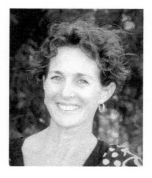

integrated system that flows naturally from regular practice into daily life through every step we take. SONW helps me feel grounded, healthy, strong, connected, calm, present and joyful. With the clarity that comes from regular SONW practice I seem to make better choices around what to eat, say and even do. SONW has been a blessing for me and I would love you to feel and experience the benefits too.

*Email: jomoloney@natural-walking.com*
*Mobile: +61400693731*

## Tanya Ulchenko, Moscow, Russia

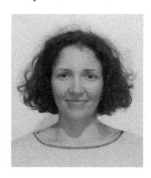

I'm a former Pilates instructor who discovered that Secrets of Natural Walking® is much easier and gives a lot more to me and my students within a single practice than any other fitness routine. SONW is a gentle, whole-body realignment, toning and moving patterns in harmony with natural gravity. SONW also offers deep cleansing and healing right down to the roots of problems (both physical and non-physical), filling us with pure energy and beneficial realizations about all the possible ways we treat our bodies.

One of my SONW students who couldn't climb the stairs unassisted for several months after a knee-replacement operation was amazed at how regular SONW practice allowed her to walk normally again after a knee replacement. Much healthier pregnancy, healed back and neck pain, better business decision-making, clearer mind are just a few awesome benefits of SONW that I witnessed.

As for me, Secrets of Natural Walking® won my heart right at my first workshop. I liked the ease and whole-body freshness it gave me, so I enjoyed it whenever I felt I needed it. Later, it took a sudden and unexpected health problem for me to become amazed at SONW's deep healing effect. I had a terrible heart rhythm for about 3 months due to stress. Every third beat felt like a huge kick in my chest. I was scared. I followed my doctor's advice and took medication, but nothing helped. Finally, I had more free time and decided to become more dedicated to SONW. I started a daily practice of 1,5 hours straight, and in only one week, my heart rate returned to normal!

Practice walking the way we are designed - and the rest will follow. So, nearby friends, feel free to contact me for a chat or a step. We are all meant to help each other and walk through this beautiful life together.

*Languages: Russian, English*
*Phone Number: +7 925 4383698*
*E-mail address: tatiana.russia@natural-walking.com*
*Whatsapp: +7 914 3207380*
*Skype: awesomehome*
*Facebook: www.facebook.com/naturalwalkingrussia*
*Instagram: naturalwalking_russia*

**Tanja Borkowski, Hamburg, Germany**
I love to practice SONW because it is my full workout for a

day. I can practice at home or with others. I am still in shape at the age of 48, and I do always look so much more relaxed when I have practiced SONW. My sleep got so great again (I had problems with it before but now it's gone!)

I love seeing how fast my SONW students' mood changes in the middle of the workshop or during practice with them: they become more open, happier/more joyful during SONW practice, and it is clear everyone experiences a better sense of well-being. It's truly beautiful to witness.

SONW is so helpful, especially if you are not joyful in your daily life, or especially if you have physical problems. For example, when you have back problems or do not feel comfortable in your body, SONW can help you so much. It is one of the best things that happened in my life, that I am able to walk properly now.

*Phone:*   *+49-1715084160*
*Email:*   *t.borkowski@natural-walking.com*
          *t.borkowski@natürliches-gehen.de*
*Web:*    *www.natürliches-gehen.de*

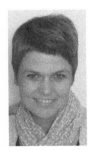

**Yvonne, Stuttgart, Germany**
SONW is a very special gift.
After a short period of practicing SONW, my daily life became lighter and happier in a very natural way. And this feeling has remained with me until today. I am also very grateful to witness the significant positive impact SONW has on the lives of many others on the emotional and the physical level. Also in cases where the traditional medicine couldn't help. My wish for you

would be that you too will have the chance to experience this special gift one day.

*Email: yvonne.kury@gmail.com*
*Phone: +49-174-3314115*

## Judy Chew, Singapore

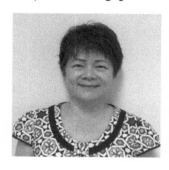

I have yet to come across any exercise that is as holistic and complete as Secrets of Natural Walking® (SONW). It has improved my physical, emotional and mental well-being greatly. SONW is easy to learn and most importantly, it is suitable for everyone, regardless of age and health. All it needs is for you to be willing to take that first step to reclaim your body and health.

I've benefitted greatly from SONW:

1) the chronic pain in my left knee is now completely gone;
2) my leg muscles feel stronger;
3) the yin-and-yang balance in my body feel balanced and aligned;
4) I have better and improved immunity; and
5) overall, my body feels much lighter – I'm able to walk longer distances and climb stairs without difficulty

As an SONW Instructor, I have also witnessed the miracles of SONW on my students. I've had a hearing-impaired participant tell me that he no longer has his gout issue bothering him. Another participant who used to suffer from chronic back aches is now able to walk around with a straight and pain-free back. Many other seniors who have participated in the SONW workshops have complimented the exercises because they feel much more revitalised and invigorated.

Come join me at the SONW workshop and experience these benefits yourself!

*Please contact me for English/Chinese SONW workshops and/or*
*introductory talk:*
*Phone: +65-97113576*
*Email: judy.chew@natural-walking.com*
*WhatsApp: +65-97113576*
*Facebook: Natural Walking – Singapore*
*Language: English/Mandarin*

## Julie Lin, Singapore

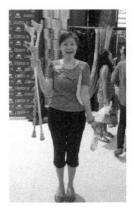

*Picture: Julie Lin freed from her crutches after SONW workshop*

Through personal experience, I have learned that nothing compares with natural healing. We are all born with natural healing abilities. The Secrets of Natural Walking® (SONW) enable us to reawaken our own body's natural healing abilities that has the most amazing healing to our whole well-being, way beyond my expectations.

I was on crutches for about a year. 5 specialists (including a TCM doctor who specializes in sport injuries and even a neurologist who prescribed nerve-pain/depression medicine and advised surgery with no guarantee to complete recovery) had given up on me, commented that my foot problem was too complicated.

After SONW Level 2, I was able to walk, but stopping the medicine had resulted in very bad withdrawal syndrome. Man-made medication provides only temporary solution, and it can have a possible danger of overly dependent and might give rise to other health issues too: not only the pain of my foot came back, my whole body, joints and muscles was all in pain. It also put me into depression, and I could not sleep even though my mind was so tired; it was a torture! Deep tissue pressure therapy was too much to bear. Not only my foot was swollen, my whole leg was swollen too!

SONW, on the other hand, is the most natural and a very simple and low-impact exercise that reaps amazing results. I started to pick up by pumping my foot while sitting, and slowly when I was able to stand up with crutches, I started to do the steps accordingly until not only am I able to walk again, all the aches and pain were gone. My mood is lifted, and I started feeling peaceful and calm. Most importantly, I can have quality sleep. My whole spine is straightened and realigned. My whole well-being is taken care of.
SONW has given me a new lease of life, and I am so grateful that every step I take, I am walking towards healthier and more peaceful living.

Please feel free to contact me if you have any queries or if you are interested in attending The Secrets of Natural Walking® in Singapore.

*Phone: +65-97211116*
*E-mail: julielxh168@gmail.com*

**Sally, Pennsylvania and New Jersey, U.S.A.**

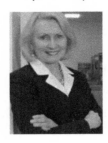

As a child, I had chronic respiratory illnesses, which continued into adult asthma. For years, I followed a routine of medical and pharmaceutical treatments. They would alleviate the symptoms for a while and then the cycle of difficulty in breathing would begin again. After practicing Secrets of Natural Walking®, I began to feel the difference in my breathing. It was freer and deeper with no tightness in the chest. My upper body posture was straighter and more relaxed. The need for my daily breathing inhaler was reduced, or sometimes not needed. I felt more energetic. My SONW students also experienced benefits from having practiced SONW. They would keep in touch about the positive changes they were experiencing. A chiropractor noted, "I'm doing the walking daily practice, seldom missing a day, and it has been very helpful. It has really helped my feet. I feel that SONW would benefit many of my patients."

My personal vision for teaching Secrets of Natural Walking® is to assist others to experience and realize, for themselves, the benefits and changes from Natural Walking on their physical body, as well as, for their mental and emotional well being. I am deeply grateful when so many share their wonderful stories of the changes they are experiencing, each unique for his or her individual needs...all happening naturally. I invite you to experience a Natural Walking Workshop, so you too can begin your pathway to a healthier you and a deeply changing experience for your whole being.

*Phone/Text/WhatsApp: +1 215-520-0192*
*Email: smydlowec@me.com*

### Gloria Brennan, Buffalo, New York, U.S.A.

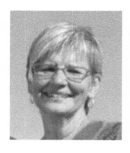

I am a true believer of the power of Natural Walking because of the results I have witnessed in myself and in the people who have taken the workshop. A 16-year-old boy with scoliosis couldn't stop smiling because he was standing straighter and hearing his grandmother say he was three inches taller. A woman cried out in joy because her chronic ankle pain was gone before we finished practicing the first key. An older gentleman said he felt like he had an invisible brace supporting his weak and painful knees. Others reported less joint and back pain, better balance and posture, more energy, and other improvements. I myself have had significant straightening and strengthening of my legs and feet, elimination of pain in my hips and back, improvement in my eyesight, and toning of my calf, thigh, chest, and stomach muscles. I, like other attendees, feel so much better physically, emotionally and spiritually. I am very grateful for the opportunity to teach the Secrets of Natural Walking® so others can feel and be so much better.

*Phone: 1 (716) 713-2152*
*Whatsapp: 1 716 713 2152*
*Email: gloria@natural-walking.com*

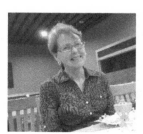

### Donna Roller, Houston and Sugar Land, TX, U.S.A.

I live in the country, so to speak, about 20 miles south of SW Houston, Texas, on some property that my husband and I share with two cats, and various wild creatures, including deer, opossum, raccoons, armadillos, and a pair of owls. When I started learning how to walk naturally with SONW, it was difficult to practice because so many parts of my body were in agony. But what I found was that if I kept practicing, all my complaints began to disappear. As my body was changing, I began to feel better – healthier and happier.

It is now clear to me that learning Secrets of Natural Walking® is the best way to take care of ourselves. The benefits affect not only our physical body, but also our mind, and our spiritual connection. As we become healthier and happier, the other people in our lives also benefit. When I teach, I remind the participants that healing takes time. Sometimes, however, it happens right away. In the last workshop, for example, one woman was standing tall and smiling, and reported the pain in her knee she had been living with was gone (after practicing for only 45 minutes).

I recommend these workshops to as many people as I can. Those that are interested in helping their bodies, minds, and spirits in a completely natural way, always find the answers they are looking for in the peace and calming that comes from just taking a simple step, slowly and deliberately, over and over. Join us. Learn to be well so you, too, can experience living healthier and happier.

*Phone:  1-281-703-6352*
*Email:  Donna@natural-walking.com*
*DonnaRoller@yahoo.com*

**Lina, Houston, Texas, U.S.A.**
I have been attending Secret of Natural Walking ever since it was first introduced in the USA. I was surprised that SONW

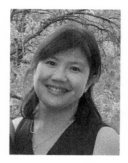

helped me feel more energized, healthier, calmer, and happier right away. Also, after doing SONW for 21 consecutive day, my blood count, which had always been low because I have been chronic anemic since I was young, was record high at the end of the 21-Day Challenge. This experience made me feel excited, and I wanted to share to more and more people.

I signed up and joined the SONW instructor team. I share, help and cheer my family and people around me to do SONW practice together whenever and wherever I can. I really enjoy supporting and helping the group practice here in Houston. As time went by, results from others started to show. I witnessed some miraculous transformation from people in the group: no more knee pain, no more frozen shoulder, no more constipation, body getting slimmer and more toned, less lower back pain, better sleep quality, better body posture, etc.

SONW gives real result! It helps people of all ages. I feel very blessed and grateful to be given the opportunity to share and teach Secret of Natural Walking to help others. This is really a Gift of Love from the Creator.

*Phone:* +18323166355
*Email:* marcelinas@yahoo.com
       onw.houston@gmail.com
*Facebook: Natural Walking - SONW Houston TX*

## Martha Luz, U.S.A.

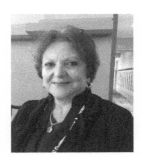

Hello! My name is Martha Luz but most people know me by my nickname: Taluza. Seeing the wonderful results that SONW has had on the people I have taught and from personal experience I can share that it helps participants to know, appreciate and feel more comfortable and relaxed with their bodies and experience less pain and stiffness. I have seen severe scoliosis been restored. I have seen cancer patients going through their treatments and surgeries and rebounding to a state of well-being that I consider miraculous. I have seen how SONW helps reduce stress, improve emotional well-being and lift the fogginess of the brain bringing about better attention, concentration, and clarity of mind. It also establishes an amazing and empowering connection to the earth and your spiritual heart.

SONW was difficult for me in the beginning: my body hurt and felt stiff and uncomfortable, but even the first time, I could feel a sense of relief and deep calmness. I was stiff and a little sore but for some reason, I knew it was good. I was tired but at the same time felt stronger and with more energy. I have become passionate and embrace SONW as with the regular practice, it continues improving and making me feel more at home in the body, and also has helped to reinforce within me, a beautiful space of peace and calmness that keeps me relaxed and grounded despite the tumult and busyness of my life. I can feel my stance and my walking becoming lighter and the stiffness so often experienced slowly disappearing, I feel younger and have a sense of well-being and contentment that I had forgotten.

I invite you to join the Secrets of Natural Walking® (SONW) workshops and daily practices. Send me an email to be added to our mailing list and I will provide you with information about classes, workshops, and practices plus if you are in my vicinity, an in-person free evaluation of your walking.

I teach SONW in Spanish, English & Portuguese in the US and in Latin America. In the US I teach in Maryland, Virginia, Washington DC, as well as in the Boston, MA areas.
In Latin America, I teach in Panama, Peru, Uruguay, and soon in Ecuador, Colombia and Guatemala.

*For the US Workshops please contact me at:*
*sonw.taluza@gmail.com*
*For information about Latin America Workshops:*
*Email: latinamerica.nwl2018@gmail.com*
*Tel: +1 240-381-8322*

**Tina Encheva, Las Vegas, Nevada, U.S.A.**
Tina teaches SONW workshops in English and in Bulgarian.
Dear Readers:
I would like to congratulate you on taking the first step to learn about Secrets of Natural Walking®. Natural Walking had profoundly changed my health and overall well-being so I would like to welcome you to our community. For many years I have suffered from lower back pain; I tried countless treatments available but the pain would come back again over time. I was so tired and over stressed that I couldn't sleep well every night.

After I practiced the six simple keys to Natural Walking, not only the pain in my lower back permanently disappeared, but I also noticed that I have a lot of energy, and I had more restful nights.

Before learning about Natural Walking, I was also treated for migraine headaches, which I would have for three to four days in a row, with me two to three times a month taking five different pills. After practicing Natural Walking consistently every day, my migraine headaches never came back to this day, and I no longer take pills.

My goal now is to educate everyone about the benefits of Secrets of Natural Walking® in our community and to organize more events where we can share and learn how to become healthier, happier, and more joyful. I hope you will find this book interesting and don't stop there, after reading it. Please continue to look for natural ways of living that will improve your health and well-being.

Happy Walking.

*Email: tina@natural-walking.com*
*Phone: 702-292-1156*
*Web: http://www.meetup.com/Secrets-of-Natural-Walking-Las-Vegas-Meetup/*

**Tim Johnson, Bournemouth, UK.**

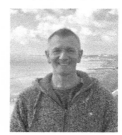

SONW removed persistent lower back pain that had been caused by years of walking incorrectly. In addition to pain elimination, I feel lighter and happier when I am walking during the day. Students have also reported many changes to their health and wellbeing.

One individual even avoided having to have a second hip operation as the changes from SONW practice corrected long-term poor walking habits.

There is nothing to lose with SONW except bad habits that have affected our health negatively for many years.

*Phone:  +44 (0)7767 775 901*
*Email:   tjse9@icloud.com*

## Caroline McCullagh, Maidenhead, London & South East, UK

In SONW, everything happens in a gentle yet thorough manner. There is a release of tension from within that is deeply relaxing and soothing, and there is also a sense that every part within is corresponding to every movement so that the body as whole is becoming re-aligned and completely well again, refreshed, toned, strong and healthy.

Many SONW students I taught have been astounded by the way they have become calm and deeply peaceful, naturally and instantly, after learning the keys of natural walking. I would encourage anyone to try it to experience for themselves how amazing it is to finally be able to fully appreciate the human body.

*Email:   sonwgb@gmail.com*
*Mobile:  +44 (0)7984936767*
*Facebook: Secrets of Natural Walking England*

## Deborah Ballon, Canada and Latin America.

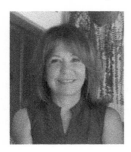

Personally, I experienced a remarkable increase in energy, both physically and mentally. My health was good, but a deep sense of wellbeing and vitality is now present throughout my entire day, along with joy in my heart, serenity and peace of mind. I constantly see striking changes on my workshop participants, from long standing health issues vastly improved, to debilitating injuries that are all but gone, and even childbirth beautifully experienced. All just by walking --naturally. I truly feel Natural Walking will touch you in a very special way, as it has touched me and so many others. It is a wonderful opportunity and you are warmly invited to join!

*Email:  ballonc@rogers.com*

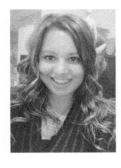

## Selina, Calgary, Canada

I feel embraced by the miracles of SONW almost every single day, from the most amazing gentle and natural shifts in my body posture and alignment, to the gentle, natural and aligning shifts in my life as a whole. On days when I practice SONW, I find that the day is easier and whatever I need seems to come to me with ease without my even having to identify those needs. So much more is accomplished in a natural and effortless way. I feel calm and joyful with a lightness and spark that also creates happiness in those around me. I feel a flow and synchronicity in my life. Over the long-term, I have found that when I am consistent in my SONW practice, solutions have sometimes come easily into my life for health concerns which I had been seeking answers to for a long time without any luck - it was like the answers came and found me. As a result, sometimes SONW has improved my health and well-being directly and at other times, SONW has sometimes cleared whatever was blocking the solutions to the health concerns, thereby allowing the solution to come effortlessly.

I have so much gratitude for the amazing ways in which SONW has transformed my life and the life of those around me that I feel very happy every time someone new signs up for their first SONW workshop because I know this is going to be the beginning of so many special changes in their life. I look forward to hearing all about the beautiful shifts you experience with SONW as a special addition in your life. I would love to meet you and share in this next phase of your journey.

*Email: selina.naturalwalking@gmail.com*

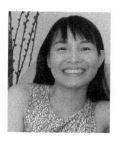

**Nancy Lim, Malaysia**
Nancy teaches SONW not only in English language but also in Bahasa Indonesia in Kuala Lumpur, Malaysia. I love the simple steps in SONW to make me healthier and happier. Call me to find out how SONW can help you or just to say hello :)

*Phone: +6019 320 2252*
*Email: limpengbeng@gmail.com*
*Languages: English, Bahasa Indonesia*

## Sandra Zein, Hong Kong

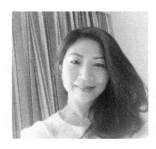

Natural walking has always been my favourite activity in the morning; a getaway from a busy life. Before I was introduced to Secrets of Natural Walking®, I used to eat a lot of "junk" foods: cake, chips, candy, you name it. However, after practising Natural Walking, my choice of food started to change - I started to opt for healthy foods. In addition, I also began to appreciate and love my body more. Natural Walking has improved my mood and my overall health; I am happier and healthier now. I am very happy to share the Secrets of Natural Walking® with you to rediscover the natural healing abilities of our bodies.

*Email: sandrazein@yahoo.com*
*Phone number: +852 91041768*
*Languages: English and Bahasa Indonesia*

## Deb LaFon, Raven, and Diana Stone teach SONW and runs SONW Center in Asheville, North Carolina, U.S.A

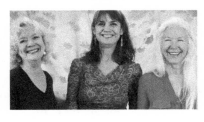

Diana Stone, Deborah Raven Kelly, Deborah La Fon are licensed instructors of Secrets of Natural Walking® and produce workshops that transform the simple act of walking into better health and well-being. Each has a personal story that brought them to their discipline. They are driven by their commitment to share Natural Walking and be part of a revolution in how people relate to their bodies and to their movement where body, mind, and heart come together. You feel good just being around this trio.

**Deb La Fon:**

I've grown to really love Natural Walking! It feels so good when my body is in proper alignment. I'm nowhere near the "old lady" I was becoming!! I can move with the strength and muscles of someone I used to know! And the adjustments happening from the soles of my feet through the energy passageways of my body are real. The sweetest joy is when I see this realization in the eyes and smiles of my students... young and old. One thing I especially love, is feeling that energetic life force in my body, knowing this is a benefit for people of every age and physical ability.

**Raven:**

Secrets of Natural Walking® has opened many doors for me to be able to live a more joyful and fulfilled life. As a former yoga instructor, I was not sure if there was much to learn here, but my eyes were opened during the first workshop I attended. I discovered muscles I didn't know existed, and have since learned how important those muscles and the energy pathways that are activated in natural walking are in helping to free our bodies and ourselves from the web of tension, stress and holding which most of us have considered "normal". This has resulted in increased energy, lighter heart, relief from chronic health issues, and much more. I witness this in both myself and in others who have attended the class and practice natural walking regularly.

Secrets of Natural Walking® is for anyone who is willing to

let go of blockages, regain their health and well-being and restore the harmony and balance that is the natural blueprint for the human body.

**Diana Stone:**

There are two things in my life that I truly feel I cannot thrive without, one is Open Heart Meditation, and the other is Natural Walking. I did not know what to expect when I first took the Natural Walking Workshop. I thought maybe the class would help me with the hiking I enjoy in the mountains nearby.

What I found in the Natural Walking class was a tool that has helped me in many aspects of my life. The most surprising one for me was psychological. I have found the Natural Walking practice to be a powerful destressor for my physical body as well as my mind. As a psychologist, this got my attention! Whenever I feel "out of whack" for whatever reason, the natural walking practice is my go-to for getting me back on center, both physically and emotionally. If I feel discomfort in my body, whether from overexertion, imbalanced use, or just tiredness, I again turn to natural walking as the remedy which works surely and very quickly, usually in minutes. I look forward to doing my natural walking practice daily as a way to feel good in all parts of my being and am grateful beyond measure for what it has given me and those I have taught.

*Email: sonwasheville@gmail.com*
*sonwasheville@natural-walking.com*
*Deb La Fon: +1 828-215-6033*
*Raven: +1 828 279-8300*
*Diana Stone: +1 828 779-4177*

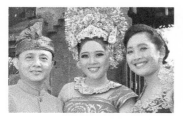

**Paramajaya (Rama) and Saraswati (Saras) teach SONW and runs SONW Center Bali Clinic, Denpasar, Bali, Indonesia**

Rama and Saras teach SONW workshops since 2014. In addition to teaching SONW workshops, we also enrich our experience and understanding about SONW and its benefits through our SONW Center in Bali. Both of us have experienced tremendous wonderful benefits from practicing SONW daily. The benefits include physical, mental, emotional and spiritual aspects. We have better vitality, stamina and joy in living our daily lives.

We have also witnessed directly how students of our workshops and members of our SONW Center experience many health benefits. Those with simple health issues to serious illness experience wonderful benefits. Some of the health issues that show significant improvements after practicing SONW regularly include influenza, stroke, vertigo, asthma, heart attack, MG (Myasthenia Gravis), knee, hips, spine and posture problems. All are simply by practicing SONW regularly. And not only the health issues reduce, the quality of their daily lives improves so much, This is possible due to the fact that our human body is an integrated system that works in harmony and with SONW regular practices, the natural healing ability of this integrated system is activated wonderfully.

At spiritual level, our heart opens more and more beautifully, giving us more joy and gratitude of having this human body as a gift of Love. We realize how wonderful this gift of Love called the human body is when we use it the way it was designed to be used. We invite you cordially to experience the joy of using our human body naturally the way it was designed through Secrets of Natural Walking®.

Rama and Saras can be reached via
*Email:*            *paramajaya@gmail.com*
                     *geksaraswati@gmail.com*
*WhatsApp/Phone:*   *+62-896-0946-1588 or*
                     *+62-811-392-5500*

**Djoko a.k.a. DJ teaches SONW and runs SONW Center in Surabaya, Java, Indonesia.**

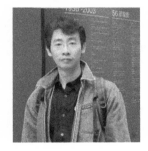

I had a pinched nerve caused by sitting improperly for long hours on airplanes. Neither acupuncture nor Qi Gong could heal me as my problem was severe: I was still in much pain. After practicing SONW for 2-3 weeks, my nerve was no longer pinched, which naturally and automatically freed me from my pain.

If you think my simple healing story is amazing, here is a healing story that amazed me: after one month of SONW practice, a 64-year-old SONW student of mine sent me photos of his ultrasound results and the letter from his doctor showing that he did not need to go into surgery for his kidney and prostate problem. He made me realize how our body truly is a beautiful Gift of Love from God and how amazing it is to get healing simply by using our body properly. By walking naturally and properly, we allow our body to heal itself, just the way it has been designed by the Creator.

In my hometown, Surabaya (in Java, Indonesia), many SONW alumni regularly get together to practice natural walking at SONW Center. So many beautiful stories have been shared amongst us. If you have any question, please feel free to contact me.

I also travel the world to teach SONW, so I may see you in your hometown.

*Email: prayinglotus@gmail.com*

## Lonneke Janosik, Yogyakarta, Indonesia

As a mother of four children I am interested in following a holistic approach to life. I always believed in the natural healing abilities of our body however it was not until my first Secret of Natural Walking (SONW/RBA) workshop that I experienced the simple keys to have these natural abilities and gifts unlocked.

I soon began to feel how my body was adjusting and realigning. The tension I had unknowingly held for so long within me, started to dissolve and my body began to function and work more like the way it had been created to. This was an amazing and wonderful feeling. It was accompanied with such a light, gentle and natural feeling of being alive in the widest sense.

Various problems with digestion and pelvic floor and slow metabolism disappeared within weeks of regular daily practice. I embraced all the physical and aesthetic benefits including my muscles becoming more toned, skin and cell rejuvenation, and the balancing of my hormones. The effects did not stop there. There was a clear and noticeable effect on my overall feeling of wellbeing. I experienced a vitality, peace and happiness that extended beyond the actual practice.

As an Open Heart Teacher and a Life Coach, I'm aware of how often people experience positive change only through a lot of effort and time. I've been amazed to see and experience how this SONW one day workshop can change people's lives so rapidly all through the simple act of doing the walking exercise daily. No special age, knowledge, ability, time, place or equipment is required! Everything you need is already within you!

Its with great excitement therefore that I share this SONW workshop with you. I teach this Workshop In English, Dutch and Indonesian worldwide. I am inviting you to join the workshop so that you too can come into alignment and unlock the great secrets just waiting to be opened and released within your body.

*Email: lonalight@yahoo.com*

# SONW Instructors' Contact Info

For the complete updated list of instructors, please go to
www.natural-walking.com/instructors

All SONW Instructors in countries where English is the
dominant language teach in English; SONW Instructors who
can teach in other languages have noted down the languages
in the table.

## AUSTRALIA

| City/State | Name | Contact Info | Languages |
|---|---|---|---|
| Alice Springs, Northern Territory | Jo Moloney | +61400693731 joeyjoinalice@gmail.com | English |
| Hobart, Tasmania | Amanda Young | +61430282073 amanda@lotuscentre.org | English |
| Hobart, Tasmania | Angela Holmes | +61421303584 akholmes@utas.edu.au | English |
| Hobart, Tasmania | Anthony Bone | +61408132562 anthony.bone9@gmail.com | English |
| Hobart, Tasmania | Cheynie Sukha | +61433324534 cheynie@natural-walking.com | English |

| Hobart,<br>Tasmania<br>Gold Coast,<br>Queensland | Georgy Michael | +61410247346<br>georgy@happyswimmers.com.au | English |
|---|---|---|---|
| Hobart,<br>Tasmania | Kent Young | +61430282048<br>kent@lotuscentre.org | English |
| Hobart,<br>Tasmania | Pat Janes | +61404854327<br>pat.h.janes@gmail.com | English |
| Melbourne,<br>Victoria | Clare Jennings | +61409385792<br>clare.jennings1@bigpond.com | English |
| Melbourne,<br>Victoria | Donna Ellerton | +61479063285<br>+61405514462<br>info@wellbodyandspirit.com | English |
| Melbourne,<br>Victoria<br>(Will travel) | Narelle Hayes | +61411607025<br>narelle@natural-walking.com | English |
| Melbourne,<br>Victoria | Nikoletta Kovacs Kha | +61437550067<br>nikikha@gmail.com | English<br>Hungarian |
| Penguin,<br>Tasmania | Gillian Brame | +61427907779<br>gillcrab64@gmail.com | English |
| Perth, Western<br>Australia | Glenn Joseph Backes | +61403257408<br>gjbackes@aol.com | English |
| Perth, Western<br>Australia | Yalda Cassidy | +61404961320<br>yaldacassidy@gmail.com | English |

| Perth, Western Australia | Sunny Tjandrakesuma | +61438510671<br>isk@iinet.net.au | English Indonesian |
|---|---|---|---|
| Perth, Western Australia | Melky Herlina | +61433919887<br>melkyherlina@gmail.com | English Indonesian |
| Perth, Western Australia | Franca Carrera | +61452225937<br>hello@francacarrera.com.au | English |
| Perth, Western Australia | Sean Holmes | +61490971966<br>sjholmes@gmail.com | English |
| Perth, Western Australia | Sheila Howes | +61410791866<br>sheh66@outlook.com | English |
| Perth, Western Australia | Jackie Holmes | +61490921393<br>jaclydholmes@gmail.com | English |
| Sydney, New South Wales | Pipina Lazaris | +61451445885<br>padmapipina@gmail.com<br>skype:pipi421 | English Greek |

## CANADA

| City/State | Name | Contact Info | Languages |
|---|---|---|---|
| Salt Spring Island, BC Victoria, BC (will travel) | John Dunham | +16048371697<br>jrdunham@natural-walking.com<br>jrdunham@shaw.ca | English |
| Calgary, AB (will travel) | Selina Bhanji | +15872290444<br>selina.naturalwalking@gmail.com | English |

| Toronto, ON (will travel) | Deborah Ballon | +19059038225<br>deborah.ballon@gmail.com | English<br>Spanish |
| Toronto, ON (will travel) | Bernadette Halloran | +14165188677<br>bernadette@innerheartsolutions.com | English |

## GERMANY

| City | Name | Contact Info | Languages |
| --- | --- | --- | --- |
| Luneburg | Dagmar Menke | +491743232011<br>dagmar.menke@gmx.de | English<br>German |
| Hamburg | Gisela Spangenberg | +491748710071<br>gisela.spangenberg@icloud.com | English<br>German |
| Hamburg | Kathrin Dworatzek | +491788854578<br>kasia.d@web.de | English<br>German |
| Hamburg | Katharina Wolf-Grünfeld | +491708067966<br>katwog@gmail.com | English<br>German |
| Stuttgart, Munich, Cologne | Yvonne Kury | +491743314115<br>yvonne.kury@gmail.com | English<br>German |
| Stuttgart, Munich | Tuan Minh Nguyen | +491729335959<br>lotusminh@gmail.com | English<br>German<br>Vietnamese |

# HONG KONG

| City | Name | Contact Info | Languages |
|---|---|---|---|
| Hong Kong | Sandra Zein | +85291041769<br>sandazein@yahoo.com | English<br>Indonesian |
| Hong Kong<br>Taiwan | Laura Fan | +15105012925<br>lfan18@yahoo.com | English<br>Chinese<br>Mandarin<br>/Cantonese |

# IRELAND

| City | Name | Contact Info | Languages |
|---|---|---|---|
| Cork, Dublin,<br>Kerry, Waterford,<br>Wexford<br>(will travel) | Darragh O'Sullivan | +353877842848<br>darragh@upwardsireland.com | English<br>Irish |
| Clare, Limerick,<br>Galway,<br>Tipperary, Kildare<br>Meath, Mayo,<br>Dublin,<br>(will travel) | Geraldine Tobin | +353874170764<br>geraldine.naturalwalking@gmail.com | English |

# INDONESIA

| City/State | Name | Contact Info | Languages |
|---|---|---|---|
| Bandung | Betty, S.E. | +62818209500<br>betty@natural-walking.com | Indonesian<br>English |
| Bandung | dr. Yelica Rachmat, S.H., M.M., MH. Kes., SpPD | +6281394336420<br>dr_yelica@yahoo.com | Indonesian<br>English |
| Bandung | Elis Tanizar | +6281809261137<br>elistanizar@gmail.com | Indonesian |
| Bandung | Ir. Gunadi | +62811205369<br>innerfire_id@yahoo.com | Indonesian |
| Bandung | Iwan Tedjasukmana | +6289664079228<br>iwantedjasukmana@gmail.com | Indonesian |
| Bandung | Linggajanti Jahja Saputra | +62816612728<br>lingga@natural-walking.com | Indonesian<br>English |
| Batam | Djaja Roeslim | +62811700305<br>unnydjaja@yahoo.com | Indonesian |
| Bogor | Wibowo Sukamuljo | +62818723184<br>wibowo_sukamulyo@indo.net.id | Indonesian |
| Denpasar | AAA Saraswati AP, S.Kom. | +628113925500<br>geksaraswati@gmail.com | Indonesian |
| Denpasar | Ir. IGPB Paramajaya, ME (Hons) | +628124625000<br>paramajaya@gmail.com | Indonesian<br>English |
| Denpasar | Irma Triharto | +628123958899<br>irmatriharto@hotmail.com | Indonesian |
| Denpasar | Ongkowidjaja | +62811380768<br>ongkojh@hotmail.com | Indonesian<br>English |

| Denpasar | Kristiina Kytoharju | +62 8121070541 | English |
| | | kristiina@santaibali.com | Finnish |
| Depok | Dr. Erna Karim, M.Si. | +6281210973997 | Indonesian |
| | | erna_karim_ui@yahoo.com | |
| Depok | Hoppy Sylvia | +6285959494434 | Indonesian |
| | | hsbambootree@gmail.com | |
| Jakarta | Agus Wicaksono | +6281514005093 | Indonesian |
| | | sonnie93@gmail.com | |
| Jakarta | Anthony Ferdinand Pajouw | +628111967227 | Indonesian |
| | | niellodojo@gmail.com | |
| Jakarta | Britt Marsietta | +6281513301492 | Indonesian |
| | | marsieta@yahoo.com | |
| Jakarta | Fita Lie | +628998787928 | Indonesian |
| | | fita@natural-walking.com | |
| Jakarta | Gunadi Widjaja | +628111980181 | Indonesian |
| | | gndwidjaja@yahoo.co.id | |
| Jakarta | Idayanti Sudiro, S.E. | +628161104995 | Indonesian |
| | | idayanti@natural-walking.com | |
| Jakarta | Ir. Kasandra Hermawan M.M. | +62819864466 | Indonesian |
| | | kasandra.hermawan@ natural-walking.com | English |
| Jakarta | Ir. Wilarjo Kurniawan | +6281908755688 | Indonesian |
| | | wilarjo@natural-walking.com | |
| Jakarta | Karto Wiwiksana | +6281385322388 | Indonesian |
| | | karto.wiwiksana@gmail.com | |
| Jakarta | Luli Asliani | +628111633316 | Indonesian |
| | | inailsa16@yahoo.com | |

| Jakarta | Nadine Ames | +6282112621661 | Indonesian |
| | | nadine.ad.ames@gmail.com | English |
| Jakarta | Olivia Sulistio | +62 82123131841 | Indonesian |
| | | cantingcandrakirana@gmail.com | English |
| Jakarta | Phang Agustini | +62811146627 | Indonesian |
| | | alexatini@yahoo.co.id | |
| Jakarta | Sangeeta Jaggia | +6281586000912 | English |
| | | sangeetajaggia@gmail.com | |
| Jakarta | Santoso Djajadi Sadikin, S. Kom. | +628128255050 | Indonesian |
| | | santosdoang@gmail.com | |
| Jakarta | Sanuk Tandon | +628119998286 | Indonesian |
| | | sanuktandon@gmail.com | English |
| Jakarta | Sjiapin Chandra | +62816886794 | Indonesian |
| | | sjiapin.chandra@ natural-walking.com | |
| Jakarta | Willy Iskandar | +6281586047075 | Indonesian |
| | | uwi@cbn.net.id | English |
| Jakarta | Yuliantie Rachman | +628129239345 | Indonesian |
| | | yuliantie_rachman@yahoo.com | |
| Karanganyar | Yunita Mubyarti | +62 811299698 | Indonesian |
| | | yunitamubyarti@gmail.com | |
| Makassar | Deane Anthony | +6285101470583 | Indonesian |
| | | deanesaja@gmail.com | |
| Makassar | Eveline Maria Philips | +6287840655044 | Indonesian |
| | | eveline_philips@yahoo.com | |
| Makassar | Satrya Purnadewi | +6281280295146 | Indonesian |
| | | dewi.satrya@gmail.com | |

| Makassar | Tjokorda Istri Sri Darmasenadi | +6285101739332<br>tjok_yuni@yahoo.com | Indonesian |
|---|---|---|---|
| Malang | Silvi Soetikno | +6281365358589<br>silvi@natural-walking.com | Indonesian<br>English |
| Medan | Andry Susanto | +628126015365<br>adt.pro99@gmail.com | Indonesian |
| Medan | Aunona | +6282226861117<br>aunona76@yahoo.com | Indonesian |
| Medan | Dewi Christianty | +628126015365<br>dewi_christianty@hotmail.com | Indonesian |
| Medan | Elly Norman | +62 812 6515651<br>ellynorman22@gmail.com | Indonesian |
| Medan | Irene Tjoatja Widjaja, S.E. | +628126031890<br>irene_mtp@yahoo.com | Indonesian |
| Medan | Nani Wong | +62811658969<br>naniwong66@yahoo.com | Indonesian |
| Medan | Soepian Junus | +62811656636<br>soepianjunus@gmail.com | Indonesian |
| Medan | Soeryanto Surya | +6282370730203<br>soeryantosurya@yahoo.com | Indonesian |
| Medan | Vincent Soenarjo | +6281808462368<br>darksquall@gmail.com | Indonesian |
| Medan | Wagiman Tandun | +62811616619<br>wagi@natural-walking.com | Indonesian<br>English |
| Medan | Yudo Surianto | +6281361648556<br>yudo_shanti@yahoo.co.id | Indonesian |
| Palembang | Felen Hidayat | +628127124277<br>felen@natural-walking.com | Indonesian |

| Palembang | Rusmala Dewy | +6281958588896 rusmaladewy@gmail.com | Indonesian |
|---|---|---|---|
| Pekanbaru | Vylonalitza | +62 811 759879 lonaarbi@gmail.com | Indonesian |
| Salatiga | Dian Anastasia Chrysanthie | +6281914349111 dian.padmagroup@yahoo.com | Indonesian |
| Samarinda | Ir. R. Ay. Esti Wahyuni, M.Si. | +6281254349394 esti.wyn@gmail.com | Indonesian |
| Samarinda | Hubertus Kusbandriyo | +6281253157459 ksbndry@yahoo.com | Indonesian |
| Semarang | Dian Widianti | +61811278551 danniwidi@yahoo.com | Indonesian |
| Surabaya | Djoko Arifin Santosa | +6281235667838 prayinglotus@gmail.com | Indonesian English |
| Surabaya | dr. Nurlaita Hartono. M.S., AAK | +628123184569 nurlaita@hotmail.com | Indonesian |
| Surabaya | I Wayan Dani Kurniawan | +6281938562885 wayandani@gmail.com | Indonesian |
| Surabaya | Yenny Hendrawati | +62811323786 yen.rba@gmail.com | Indonesian |
| Tangerang | Yustinus Sumbogo | +6281382923535 yustinus.sumbogo@ natural-walking.com | Indonesian English |
| Yogyakarta | Lonneke Janosik | +62818250117 lonalight@yahoo.com | Indonesian English |
| Yogyakarta | Nino Susanto | +62811253792 ninosusanto@gmail.com | Indonesian English |

| Yogyakarta | Tetty Julianti | +628122709617 tettyj@natural-walking.com | Indonesian English |
|---|---|---|---|

## JAPAN

| City | Name | Contact Info | Languages |
|---|---|---|---|
| Kansai (will travel) | Rico Tanaka | +13105914121 hellohappyheart@gmail.com | English Japanese |

## LATIN AMERICA

| City | Name | Contact Info | Languages |
|---|---|---|---|
| All Latin America | Martha Luz Atkinson (Taluza) | +12403818322 latinamerica.nwl2018@gmail.com | English Portuguese Spanish |
| All Latin America | Deborah Ballon | +19059038225 deborah.ballon@gmail.com | English Spanish |
| Panama, Panama | Itzel Alvarado | +50766743198 itzelalvaradol@gmail.com | English Spanish |

## MALAYSIA

| City | Name | Contact Info | Languages |
|---|---|---|---|
| Kuala Lumpur | Nancy Lim | +60193202252 nancy.lim@natural-walking.com | English Indonesian |

## NEW ZEALAND

| City | Name | Contact Info | Languages |
|------|------|--------------|-----------|
| Auckland | Raewyn Somers | +6478320121<br>+64211345935<br>raewyn.somers@gmail.com | English |
| Hamilton, Waikato | Jane Wheeler | +64212407302<br>jane@natural-walking.com | English<br>French<br>Spanish |
| Tauranga, Napier (will travel) | Murray Sawyer | +6421578017<br>murraysawyer@gmail.com | English |

## RUSSIA

| City | Name | Contact Info | Languages |
|------|------|--------------|-----------|
| Vladivostok | Tatiana Ulchenko | +79143207380<br>awesomehome@gmail.com | English<br>Russian |

## SINGAPORE

| City | Name | Contact Info | Languages |
|------|------|--------------|-----------|
| Singapore | Chew Wai Leng Judy | +6597113576<br>judy.chew@natural-walking.com<br>reikijudy.chew@hotmail.com | English<br>Chinese |
| Singapore | Lau Suan Lay (Janette) | +6597831209<br>touchedjlau@gmail.com | English |

| Singapore | Julie Lin XinHong | +6597211116<br>julielxh168@gmail.com | English<br>German |
| Singapore | Lutfiani Reed | +6583930946<br>lutfiani.reed@gmail.com | English<br>Indonesian |
| Singapore | Nancy Lim | +60193202252<br>nancy.lim@natural-walking.com | English<br>Indonesian |
| Singapore | Shinta Narulita | +6593822605<br>shinta_narulita@yahoo.co.uk | English<br>Indonesian<br>Mandarin<br>Teo Chew |

## SPAIN

| City | Name | Contact Info | Languages |
|------|------|--------------|-----------|
| Palma, Mallorca | Gerard Laracy | +34646383143<br>gerard@natural-walking.com | English<br>Spanish |

## UNITED KINGDOM

| City | Name | Contact Info | Languages |
|------|------|--------------|-----------|
| Bangor, County Down, Northern Ireland | Anastasia Ardiastuti Mcilroy | +447493196651<br>tutiardi@natural-walking.com | English<br>Indonesian |
| Bournemouth | Tim Johnson | +447767775901<br>timjohnson@natural-walking.com | English<br>German |

| Bucks, Home Counties, London | Jacqui Gascoyne | +447715171206 jacqui.naturalwalking@gmail.com | English |
| Maidenhead, London & South East (will travel) | Caroline McCullagh | +441628 417360 +447984936767 sonwgb@gmail.com | English |

## UNITED STATES

| City | Name | Contact Info | Languages |
| --- | --- | --- | --- |
| Buffalo, New York | Gloria Brennan | +17167132152 gloria@natural-walking.com | English |
| Columbia, California | Anita Read | +14102155959 anita@natural-walking.com | English |
| Los Angeles, California | Anyez Cheung | +13106631864 anyez@natural-walking.com | English |
| San Diego, California | Gayatri Burden | +19135684681 lotusheartsmiling@gmail.com | English |
| Los Angeles, California | Joe Rogers | +13106863859 joe@natural-walking.com | English |
| Los Angeles, California | Mary Hong | +13237429306 lotusHeart07@gmail.com | English |
| Chicago Milwaukee Indiana (will travel) | Rico Tanaka | +13105914121 hellohappyheart@gmail.com | English Japanese |

| Los Angeles, California | Sharon Rahmanian | +18183833633 sharon@natural-walking.com | English Farsi |
|---|---|---|---|
| Los Angeles, California | Stephanie Bloom | +13104720505 stephanie@natural-walking.com | English |
| Los Angeles, California | Kaveh Tayeban | +13108820717 lakt@hotmail.com | English Farsi |
| Los Angeles, California | Jennifer Plasencia | +19512069956 Jenplasencia@gmail.com | English Spanish |
| Mill Valley, California San Francisco Bay Area, California | John Benko | +14156023263 john_benko@yahoo.com | English |
| Southern California: Long Beach, Orange County | Joyful Linda | US.CA.Linda@gmail.com | English Indonesian |
| California, Walnut Creek, All San Francisco Bay Area, Sacramento New Jersey, North Carolina, Raleigh Durham | Laura Fan | +15105012925 lfan18@yahoo.com | English Chinese Mandarin /Cantonese |
| Maryland, Virginia, Washington DC & Boston, MA | Martha Luz Atkinson (Taluza) | +12403818322 sonw.taluza@gmail.com | English Spanish Portuguese |

| | | | |
|---|---|---|---|
| Amherst, New York | Anne Egan | +17164652225<br>aegan@natural-walking.com | English |
| Washington DC, Maryland, Virginia, NJ. (will travel) | Azam Babataher | +13014666570<br>a_babataher@yahoo.com<br>azam.babataher@gmail.com | English<br>Persian |
| Washington DC, Maryland, Virginia, Delaware<br><br>China | Aixia Zhang | +13019795166<br>aixia@natural-walking.com | English<br><br>Chinese<br>Mandarin<br>/Cantonese |
| Oak Hill, West Virginia | Caroline Cowdery | +14103530585<br>carolinecowdrey@hotmail.com | English |
| Berkeley, California | David Kelley | +15104995446<br>quahog.ri.dk@gmail.com | English<br>American<br>Sign<br>Language |
| Las Vegas, Nevada | Tina Encheva | +17022921156<br>tina@natural-walking.com | English<br>Bulgarian |
| Lewisburg, Pennsylvania | Crystal Sanders | +15707138340<br>crystal@natural-walking.com | English |

| Asheville, North Carolina (will travel) | Deborah La Fon | +18282156033 sonwasheville@gmail.com or sonwasheville@natural-walking.com | English |
|---|---|---|---|
| Asheville, North Carolina Atlanta, Georgia, (will travel) | Deborah "Raven" Kelly | +18282798300 sonwasheville@gmail.com or sonwasheville@natural-walking.com | English |
| Asheville, North Carolina, (will travel) | Diana Stone | +18287794177 sonwasheville@gmail.com or sonwasheville@natural-walking.com | English |
| Asheville, North Carolina | Dianna Lee | +18289630213 diannalee333@gmail.com | English |
| Boone, North Carolina | Diana Latendresse | +18287733640 diana@boonenc.org | English |
| Lansdale, PA and Ship Bottom, NJ | Gloria Carroll | +12159172307 gloriapc@aol.com | English |
| Asheville, North Carolina | Sexton | +18282427808 sexton@charter.net | English |

| San Antonio, TX | Graham Whitley | +12522868899 lotus.grahamw@gmail.com | English |
|---|---|---|---|
| Grants Pass, Oregon; Seattle, Washington; East Hartford, Connecticut; and San Diego, California | Susan Barrett | +15414792046 +16192487704 SueBarrett@natural-walking.com ob440sb61@gmail.com | English |
| Pennsylvania New Jersey | Sally Mydlowec | +12155200192 smydlowec@me.com | English |
| Houston, Texas Sugar Land, TX | Donna Roller | +12817036352 donna@natural-walking.com donnaroller@yahoo.com | English |
| Houston, Texas | Lina Sidik | +18323166355 marcelinas@yahoo.com or sonw.houston@gmail.com | English Indonesian |
| Washington, DC, Maryland, Virginia, (will travel) | Patricia Lee | +12024877533 itspleemail@yahoo.com | English |

# Irmansyah Effendi M.Sc.
# Book List

1.  *Smile to your heart: Simple Meditations for Peace, Health and Spiritual Growth*, 2010
2.  *Real You: Beyond Forms and Lives*, 2012
3.  Kundalini: Teknik Efektif untuk Membangkitkan, Membersihkan dan Memurnikan Kekuatan Luar Biasa dalam Diri Anda, 1998. (In Indonesian) *Kundalini: An Effective Technique to Awaken, Cleanse and Purify the Extraordinary Power within*, 1998
4.  Reiki: Teknik Efektif untuk Membangkitkan Kemampuan Penyembuhan Luar Biasa Secara Seketika, 1999. (In Indonesian) *Reiki: An Effective Technique to Instantaneously Awaken a Powerful Healing Ability*, 1999
5.  Reiki 2: Pemantapan dan Pemanfaatan dalam Hidup Sehari-hari, 1999. (In Indonesian) *Reiki 2: Mastering and Practicing in Daily Life*, 1999
6.  Lima Gerakan Awet Muda Tibet (Edisi Revisi): Teknik Efektif untuk Meraih Kebugaran, Mempertahankan Keremajaan, dan Menghambat Proses Penuaan, 2012. (In Indonesian) *Five Rejuvenating Tibetan Movements (Revised Edition): An Effective Technique to Reach Fitness, Maintaining Youth and Stopping the Ageing Process*, 2012
7.  Kundalini 2: Pendalaman dan Teknik Lanjutan, 2000. (In Indonesian) *Kundalini 2: A Deeper Discussion and More Advanced Techniques*, 2000

8. Reiki Tummo: Teknik Efektif untuk Meningkatkan Kesadaran dan Energi Spiritual, 2001. (In Indonesian) *Reiki Tummo: An Effective Technique to Increase Awareness and Spiritual Energy, 2001*

9. Hati Nurani, 2002. (In Indonesian) *Inner Heart, 2002*

10. Mencapai Tujuan Hidup yang Sebenarnya, 2003. (In Indonesian) *Attaining the True Purpose of Life, 2003*

11. Reiki Tummo: An Effective Technique for Health and Happiness, 2004

12. Seri Hati dan Kasih: Akal Budi, 2007 (In Indonesian) *Heart and Love Series: Mind and Conscience, 2007*

13. *Heart and Love Series: Sweetheart, 2007* (Translation in English from Indonesian)

14. *Serie Herz und Liebe: Süsse Herz, 2007* (Translation in German from Indonesian)

15. *Serie Corazon y Amor: Dulce Corazon, 2008* (Translation in Spanish from Indonesian)

16. Hati: Mengenal, membuka dan memanfaatnya, 2013 (Revised Edition) (In Indonesian) *Heart: Getting Acquainted, Opening and Benefiting from and Open Heart*

17. Menuai Hasil dalam Reiki: Teknik Mengoptimalkan Energi Reiki Secara Luar Biasa, 2009 (In Indonesian) *Reaping Results in Reiki: A Technique to Optimize Reiki Energy Extraordinarily, 2009*

18. Kesadaran Jiwa: Teknik Efektif untuk Mencapai Kesadaran yang Lebih Tinggi (Revisi Tambahan: Metode Perpindahan Kesadaran), 1999, 2009. (In Indonesian) *Soul Consciousness: An Effective Technique to Reach your Higher Consciousness (Additional Revision: Consciousness Shifting Method), 1999, 2009*

19. Shing Chi: Teknik Efektif untuk Mengakses Energi Ilahi (Edisi Revisi), 2009 (In Indonesian) *Shing Chi: An Effective Technique to Access Divine Energy (Revised Edition), 2009*

20. Rahasia Berjalan Alami: Aktifkan Kemampuan Penyembuhan Luar Biasa Tubuh Anda, 2016 (In Indonesian) *Secrets of Natural Walking® (SONW): Activate the Extraordinary Healing Capabilities of Your Body, 2016*

# Thank You

In addition to my deepest gratitude to True Source for all the Gifts of Love I have received in completing this book that it may reach all of you, I also wish to take this opportunity to express my appreciation to the following individuals for their contributions:

- Enrico Iskandar for translating this book
- Krissan Iskandar for providing the illustrations and formatting of this book
- dr. Yelica for giving comments and proofreading and editing this book
- dr. Roys and dr. Julius for giving comments for this book
- Printers and distributors for this book

# About the Writer

Irmansyah Effendi graduated with a Bachelor of Science in Computer Science and Mathematics at the age of 20 with magna cum laude and honor from California State University, United States. He graduated with a Master of Science, majoring in Computer Science and specializing in Artificial Intelligence at the age of 21 from the same university.

After reaching his true self consciousness, he realized how Divine Source loves and takes care of all beings completely, always wants to help, guide, and give the best. That are the ones who are still too busy with our own wants and personal needs. He realised that in praying to Divine Source, we are usually busy with our wants and needs and not using our heart or inner heart. He also understood that we usually remember and pray to Divine Source, not for Divine Source, but for ourselves, for instance to go to heaven, for our earthly needs, etc.

After this, Irmansyah introduced Open Heart prayer, which is non-denominational. Open Heart prayer invites everyone to strengthen and open their hearts to Divine Source so that they can realize more clearly how Divine Source really loves and takes care of us all and so that they can trust and surrender more to Divine Source allowing Divine Source Love to give us the most beautiful and wonderful things on earth and the afterlife. Irmansyah Effendi has shared with thousands worldwide that prosperity, health and joy are all part of Divine Source unlimited gifts of love for you, and we need to remember that our lives are just facilities to be closer to Divine Source.

CPSIA information can be obtained
at www.ICGtesting.com
Printed in the USA
FFHW021126250919
55181465-60926FF